Lecture Notes in Computer Science 9958

Commenced Publication in 1973
Founding and Former Series Editors:
Gerhard Goos, Juris Hartmanis, and Jan van Leeuwen

Editorial Board

More information about this series at http://www.springer.com/series/7412

Raj Shekhar · Stefan Wesarg
Miguel Ángel González Ballester
Klaus Drechsler · Yoshinobu Sato
Marius Erdt · Marius George Linguraru
Cristina Oyarzun Laura (Eds.)

Clinical Image-Based Procedures

Translational Research in Medical Imaging

5th International Workshop, CLIP 2016
Held in Conjunction with MICCAI 2016
Athens, Greece, October 17, 2016
Proceedings

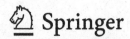 Springer

Editors

Raj Shekhar
Children's National Health System
Washington, DC
USA

Yoshinobu Sato
NAIST
Nara
Japan

Stefan Wesarg
Fraunhofer IGD
Darmstadt
Germany

Marius Erdt
Fraunhofer IDM@NTU
Singapore
Singapore

Miguel Ángel González Ballester
ICREA - Universitat Pompeu Fabra
Barcelona
Spain

Marius George Linguraru
Children's National Health System
Washington, DC
USA

Klaus Drechsler
Fraunhofer IGD
Darmstadt
Germany

Cristina Oyarzun Laura
Fraunhofer IGD
Darmstadt
Germany

ISSN 0302-9743   ISSN 1611-3349 (electronic)
Lecture Notes in Computer Science
ISBN 978-3-319-46471-8   ISBN 978-3-319-46472-5 (eBook)
DOI 10.1007/978-3-319-46472-5

Library of Congress Control Number: 2016934443

LNCS Sublibrary: SL6 – Image Processing, Computer Vision, Pattern Recognition, and Graphics

Printed on acid-free paper

This Springer imprint is published by Springer Nature
The registered company is Springer International Publishing AG
The registered company address is: Gewerbestrasse 11, 6330 Cham, Switzerland

Preface

On October 17, 2016, The International Workshop on Clinical Image-Based Procedures: From Planning to Intervention (CLIP 2016) was held in Athens, Greece, in conjunction with the 19th International Conference on Medical Image Computing and Computer-Assisted Intervention (MICCAI). Following the tradition set in the last four years, this year's edition of the workshop was as productive and exciting a forum for the discussion and dissemination of clinically tested, state-of-the-art methods for image-based planning, monitoring, and evaluation of medical procedures as in yesteryears.

Over the past few years, there has been considerable and growing interest in the development and evaluation of new translational image-based techniques in the modern hospital. For a decade or more, a proliferation of meetings dedicated to medical image computing has created the need for greater study and scrutiny of the clinical application and validation of such methods. New attention and new strategies are essential to ensure a smooth and effective translation of computational image-based techniques into the clinic. For these reasons and to complement other technology-focused MICCAI workshops on computer-assisted interventions, the major focus of CLIP 2016 was on filling gaps between basic science and clinical applications.

Members of the medical imaging community were encouraged to submit work centered on specific clinical applications, including techniques and procedures based on clinical data or already in use and evaluated by clinical users. Once again, the event brought together world-class researchers and clinicians who presented ways to strengthen links between computer scientists and engineers and surgeons, interventional radiologists, and radiation oncologists.

In response to the call for papers, 16 original manuscripts were submitted for presentation at CLIP 2016. Each of the manuscripts underwent a meticulous double-blind peer review by three members of the Program Committee, all of them prestigious experts in the field of medical image analysis and clinical translations of technology. A member of the Organizing Committee further oversaw the review of each manuscript. In all, 62 % of the submissions (i.e., 10 manuscripts) were accepted for oral presentation at the workshop. The accepted contributors represented eight countries from four continents: Europe, North America, Asia, and Australia. The three highest-scoring manuscripts were nominated to compete for the best paper award at the workshop. The final standing (first, second, and third) will be determined by votes cast by workshop participants, excluding the workshop organizers. The three nominated papers are:

- "Personalized Optimal Planning for the Surgical Correction of Metopic Craniosynostosis," by Antonio R. Porras, Dženan Zukić, Andinet Equobahrie, Gary F. Rogers, Marius George Linguraru, from the Children's National Health System in Washington, DC, USA
- "Validation of an Improved Patient-Specific Mold Design for Registration of In-Vivo MRI and Histology of the Prostate," by An Elen, Sofie Isebaert, Frederik

De Keyzer, Uwe Himmelreich, Steven Joniau, Lorenzo Tosco, Wouter Everaerts, Tom Dresselaers, Evelyne Lerut, Raymond Oyen, Roger Bourne, Frederik Maes, Karin Haustermans, from the University of Leuven, Belgium

- "Stable Anatomical Structure Tracking for Video-Bronchoscopy Navigation," by Antonio Esteban Lansaque, Carles Sanchez, Agns Borrs, Antoni Rosell, Marta Diez-Ferrer, Debora Gil, from the Universitat Autonoma de Barcelona, Spain.

We would like to congratulate warmly all the nominees for their outstanding work and wish them best of luck for the final competition. We would also like to thank our sponsor, MedCom, for their support.

Judging by the contributions received, CLIP 2016 was a successful forum for the dissemination of emerging image-based clinical techniques. Specific topics include various image segmentation and registration techniques, applied to various part of the body. The topics further range from interventional planning to navigation of devices and navigation to the anatomy of interest. Clinical applications cover the skull, the cochlea, cranial nerves, the aortic valve, wrists, and the abdomen, among others. We also saw a couple of radiotherapy applications this year. The presentations and discussions around the meeting emphasizes current challenges and emerging techniques in image-based procedures, strategies for clinical translation of image-based techniques, the role of computational anatomy and image analysis for surgical planning and interventions, and the contribution of medical image analysis to open and minimally invasive surgery.

As always, the workshop featured two prominent experts as keynote speakers. Underscoring the translational, bench-to-bedside theme of the workshop, Prof. Georgios Sakas of TU Darmstadt gave a talk on how to turn ideas into companies. Dr. Pavlos Zoumpoulis of Diagnostic Echotomography delivered a talk on his work related to ultrasound. We are grateful to our keynote speakers for their participation in the workshop.

We would like to acknowledge the invaluable contributions of our entire Program Committee, many members of which have actively participated in the planning of the workshop over the years, and without whose assistance CLIP 2016 would not have been possible. Our thanks also go to all the authors in this volume for the high quality of their work and the commitment of time and effort. Finally, we are grateful to the MICCAI organizers for supporting the organization of CLIP 2016.

August 2016

Raj Shekhar
Stefan Wesarg
Miguel Ángel González Ballester
Klaus Drechsler
Yoshinobu Sato
Marius Erdt
Marius George Linguraru
Cristina Oyarzun Laura

Organization

Organizing Committee

Klaus Drechsler	Fraunhofer IGD, Germany
Marius Erdt	Fraunhofer IDM@NTU, Singapore
Miguel Ángel González Ballester	Universitat Pompeu Fabra, Spain
Marius George Linguraru	Children's National Health System, USA
Cristina Oyarzun Laura	Fraunhofer IGD, Germany
Yoshinobu Sato	Nara Institute of Science and Technology, Japan
Raj Shekhar	Children's National Health System, USA
Stefan Wesarg	Fraunhofer IGD, Germany

Program Committee

Mario Ceresa	Universitat Pompeu Fabra, Spain
Juan Cerrolaza	Children's National Health System, USA
Yufei Chen	Tongji University, China
Jan Egger	TU Graz, Austria
Gloria Fernández-Esparrach	Hospital Clinic Barcelona, Spain
Moti Freiman	Harvard Medical School, USA
Debora Gil	Universitat Autonoma de Barcelona, Spain
Tobias Heimann	Siemens, Germany
Weimin Huang	Institute for Infocomm Research, Singapore
Sukryool Kang	Children's National Health System, USA
Xin Kang	Sonavex Inc., USA
Yogesh Karpate	Children's National Health System, USA
Michael Kelm	Siemens, Germany
Xinyang Liu	Children's National Health System, USA
Jianfei Liu	Duke University, USA
Awais Mansoor	Children's National Health System, USA
Diana Nabers	German Cancer Research Center, Germany
Antonio R. Porras	Children's National Health System, USA
Mauricio Reyes	University of Bern, Switzerland
Carles Sanchez	Universitat Autonoma de Barcelona, Spain
Akinobu Shimizu	Tokyo University of Agriculture and Technology, Japan
Jiayin Zhou	Institute for Infocomm Research, Singapore
Stephan Zidowitz	Fraunhofer MEVIS, Germany

Sponsoring Institution

MedCom GmbH

Contents

Detection of Wrist Fractures in X-Ray Images

Raja Ebsim[1](✉), Jawad Naqvi[2], and Tim Cootes[1]

[1] The University of Manchester, Manchester, UK
{raja.ebsim,tim.cootes}@manchester.ac.uk
[2] Salford Royal Hospital, Salford, UK
naqvi.jawad@gmail.com

Abstract. The commonest diagnostic error in Accident and Emergency
(A&E) units is that of missing fractures visible in X-ray images, usually
because the doctors are inexperienced or not sufficiently expert. The most
commonly missed are wrist fractures [7,11]. We are developing a fully-
automated system for analysing X-rays of the wrist to identify fractures,
with the goal of providing prompts to doctors to minimise the number of
fractures that are missed. The system automatically locates the outline
of the bones (the radius and ulna), then uses shape and texture features to classify abnormalities. The system has been trained and tested
on a set of 409 clinical posteroanterior (PA) radiographs of the wrist
gathered from a local A&E unit, 199 of which contain fractures. When
using the manual shape annotations the system achieves classification
performance of 95.5 % (area under the Receiver Operating Characteristic (ROC) curve in cross validation experiments). In fully automatic
mode the performance is 88.6 %. Overall the system demonstrates the
potential to reduce diagnostic mistakes in A&E.

Keywords: Image analysis · Image interpretation and understanding ·
X-ray fracture detection · Wrist fractures · Radius fractures · Ulna
fractures

1 Introduction

When people visit an A&E unit, one of the commonest diagnostic errors is that
a fracture which is visible on an X-ray is missed by the clinician on duty. This
is usually because they are more junior and may not have sufficient training
in interpretting radiographs. This problem is widely acknowledged, so in many
hospitals X-rays are reviewed by an expert radiologist at a later date - however
this can lead to significant delays on missed fractures which can have an impact
on the eventual outcome.

Wrist fractures are amonst the most commonly missed. To address this we are
developing a system which can automatically analyse radiographs of the wrist in
order to identify abnormalities and thus prompt clinicians, hopefully reducing
the number of errors.

We describe a fully-automated system for detecting fractures in PA wrist
images. Using an approach similar to that in [9], a global search is performed

© Springer International Publishing AG 2016
R. Shekhar et al. (Eds.): CLIP 2016, LNCS 9958, pp. 1–8, 2016.
DOI: 10.1007/978-3-319-46472-5_1

for finding the approximate position of the wrist in the image. The outlines of the distal radius and distal ulna are located using a Random Forest Regression Voting Constrained Local Model (RFCLM) [4]. We then use features derived from the shape of the bones and the image texture to identify fractures, using a random forest classifier.

In the following we describe the system in more detail, and present results of experiments evaluating the performance of each component of the system and the utility of different choices of features. We find that if we use manually annotated points, the system can achieve a classification performance of over 95 %, measured using the area under the ROC curve (AUC) for Fracture vs Normal, showing the approach has great potential. The fully automatic system achieves a performance of 88.6 % AUC, with the loss of performance being caused by the locations of the bone outlines being less accurate. However, we believe that this can be improved with larger training sets and that the system has the potential to reduce the number of fractures missed in A&E.

2 Background

A retrospect study [7] of diagnostic errors over four years, in a busy district general hospital A&E department, reported that:

- missing the abnormality on radiographs was cause of 77.8 % of the diagnostic errors,
- fractures constituted 79.7 % of diagnostic errors
- 17.4 % of the missed fractures were wrist fractures.

In a retrospective review [11] of all radiographs over 9-year period in A&E department it was found that almost 55.8 % of the missed bone abnormalities are fractures and dislocations. Fractures in radius alone constitutes 7.9 % of the missed fractures. A study [15] about missed extremity fractures at A&E showed that wrist fractures are the most common among all extremity fractures (19.7 %) with miss rate of 4.1 %.

Fractures of the distal radius alone are estimated to be 17.5 %–18 % of the fractures seen in A&E in adults [5,6] and of 25 % of the fractures seen in A&E in children [6]. There has been an increase in the incidence of these fractures in all age groups with no clear reasons, some put this increase down to lifestyle influence, osteoporosis, child-obesity and sports- related activities [12]. A study [7] showed that 5.5 % of diagnostic errors (due to abnormality missed on radiographs) were initially misdiagnosed as sprained wrist, 42 % of which were distal radius fractures.

Previous work on detecting fractures in X-ray images has been done on a variety of anatomical regions, including arm fractures [16], femur fractures [1,8, 10,14,17], and vertebral endplates [13]. The only work we are aware of regarding detecting fractures in the wrist (i.e. distal radius) is that of [8,10] where three types of features extracted from the X-ray images: Gabor, Markov Random Field, and gradient intensity features, which were used to train SVM classifiers.

The best results that they obtained used combinations of the outputs of the SVMs. They achieved good performance (accuracy≈sensitivity≈96 %) but were working on a small dataset (only 23 fractured examples in their test set).

Others [2] explored different anatomical regions using stacked random forests to fuse different feature representations. They acheived sensitivity≈81 %, and precision≈25 %.

Fractures might be seen as random and irregular so that they can not be represented with shape models. However the medical literature shows that there are patterns according to which a bone fractures. For instance, [6] describes a list of common eponyms used in clinical practice to describe these patterns in the wrist area. We adopted these patterns in our annotations as variants of normal shape. Such statistical shape models will not only be useful for detecting obvious fractures but also for detecting more subtle fractures. Fractures cause deformities that are quantified in radiographic assessments in terms of measurements of bone geometry (i.e. angles, lengths). Slight deformities might not be noticible by eye. For this reason we do not only use shape models to segment the targeted bones, as in [8], but also for capturing these deformities.

3 Method

The outlines of the two bones constituting the wrist area (i.e. Distal Ulna, Distal Radius) were annotated with 48 points and 45 points respectively (Fig. 1). These points were used to build three different models: an ulna model, a radius model, and a wrist model (combining the two bones).

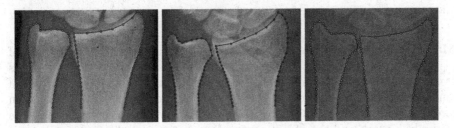

Fig. 1. The annotation on a normal wrist (left), and on wrists with an obvious fracture (middle), and a subtle fracture (right).

3.1 Modeling and Matching

The annotations are used to train a statistical shape model and an RFCLM [4] object detection model to locate the bones on new images. This step is not only needed for segmenting the targeted structures from the background but also to provide features for classification.

Building Models for Shape and Texture. The outline of each bony structure is modeled by a linear statistical shape model [3].

Each training image is annotated with n feature points. A feature point i in an image is represented by (x_i, y_i) which results in a vector x of length $2n$ representing all feature points in an image (i.e. shape vector).

$$\mathbf{x} = (x_1, ..., x_n, y_1, ..., y_n)^T \tag{1}$$

Shape vectors of all training images are aligned first to remove the variations that come from different scaling, rotation, and translation before applying principle component analysis PCA. Each shape vector $\mathbf{x}$ can be written as a linear combination of the modes of variation ($\mathbf{P}$)

$$\mathbf{x} \approx \bar{\mathbf{x}} + \mathbf{Pb} \tag{2}$$

where $\bar{\mathbf{x}}$ is the mean shape, $\mathbf{P}$ is the set of the eigenvectors corresponding to the t highest eignvalues, and $\mathbf{b}$ is the vector of the resulting shape parameters. Multivariate Gaussian probability distribution of $\mathbf{b}$ is learned from the training set. A shape is called plausible if its corresponding $\mathbf{b}$ has a probability greater than or equal some threshold probability p_t (usually set to 0.98).

Similarly, statistical texture models [3] are built by applying PCA to vectors of normalised intensity ($\mathbf{g}$) sampled from the regions defined by the points of the shape model.

$$\mathbf{g} \approx \bar{\mathbf{g}} + \mathbf{P}_g \mathbf{b}_g \tag{3}$$

The shape parameters $\mathbf{b}$ (in Eq. 2) and the texture parameters $\mathbf{b}_g$ (in Eq. 3) are used as features on which classifiers are trained to distinguish between normal and fractured bones.

Matching Shape Models on New Images. An approach similar to that of [9] is followed to locate the outline of the targeted bones. Single global model is trained to initially find approximate position of a box containing two anatomical landmarks (the Ulna styloid and Radius styloid processes). As in [9] a random forest regressor with Hough voting trained to find the displacement between the center of a patch and the object center. During training, different patches are cropped at different displacements and scales from the object center and fed to a Random Forest to learn the functional dependency between the patch's pixel intensities and the displacement. By scanning a new image at different scales and orientations with the Random Forest and collecting the votes, the most likely center, scale and orientation of the object can be found.

The box estimated by the global searcher is used to initialise a local search for the outline of the bones. We used a sequence of local searchers with models of increasing resolution. In our system, two RFCLM models are built to find the outline of wrist (i.e. two bones together), then each bone is refined separately using a sequence of four local RFCLM models.

3.2   Classification

The full automatic search gives a detailed annotation of the bony structures on each image. We trained classifiers (Random Forests with 100 trees) to distinguish between normal and fractured cases using features derived from the shape (the shape parameters, $\mathbf{b}$) and the texture (the texture model parameters, $\mathbf{b}_g$). We performed a series of cross validation experiments with different combinations of models and features.

4   Results

Data. A dataset of 409 PA radiographs of normal (210) and fractured (199) wrists was provided by a clinician at a local hospital, drawn from standard clinical images collected at the A&E unit.

Annotation. For experiments with fully automatic annotation we generated the points by dividing the set into three, training models on two subsets and applying them to the third. The mean point-to-curve distance [9] was recorded as a percentage of a reference width, then converted to mm by assuming a mean width of 25 mm, 15 mm, and 50 mm for radius, ulna, and wrist respectively. The global searcher failed in only 3 images out of 409 (i.e. 0.73 %) which are excluded in calculating the results shown in Table 1. The mean error was less than 1 mm on 95 % of the images.

Table 1. The mean point-to-curve distance in (mm) of fully automatic annotation

Shape	Mean	Median	90 %	95 %	99 %
Radius	0.35	0.29	0.62	0.78	1.23
Ulna	0.13	0.12	0.28	0.37	0.59
Wrist	0.20	0.17	0.31	0.37	0.63

Classification. We performed 5-fold cross validation experiments to evaluate which features were most useful. We use a random forest classifier (100 trees), with shape/texture model parameters as features, with (i) each bone separately, (ii) with the parameters for the bones concatenated together and (iii) the parameters from a combined wrist model of both bones together.

Table 2 shows the results of performing the classification on shape parameters alone for different bony structures expressed as area under curve AUC. The classification based on manual annotations provides an upper limit on performance, and gives encouraging results. Table 2 shows that the shape parameters of Ulna, extracted from automatic annotation, are less informative. Visual inspection of the automatic annotation suggests that the model fails to match accurately to the Ulna styloid when it is broken (Fig. 2). This leads to a drop in performance from 0.832 to 0.662 between manual and automatic results. Nevertheless, the Ulna model still contains information not captured in the Radius model which caused an improvement in results when concatenating the shape parameters of Radius and Ulna compared to the results from Radius alone.

Table 2. AUC for Classification using Shape parameters for manual and fully automated annotation

Shape	Manual	Fully automated
Radius	0.856 ± 0.008	0.816 ± 0.007
Ulna	0.832 ± 0.007	0.662 ± 0.01
Radius + Ulna	**0.926 ± 0.005**	**0.839 ± 0.01**
Wrist	0.914 ± 0.006	0.833 ± 0.004

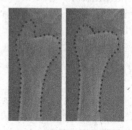

Fig. 2. Manual annotation (left) of a fractured Ula styloid process and the automatic annotation (right) that fails to locate it.

Table 3 shows classification using texture parameters, $\mathbf{b}_g$ and suggests that texture is more informative than shape and less affected by the inaccuracies in the extraction of the bone contours (See Radius results).

Table 3. AUC for Classification using Texture parameters for manual and fully automated annotation

Texture	Manual	Fully automated
Radius	0.896 ± 0.003	**0.881 ± 0.004**
Ulna	0.860 ± 0.006	0.716 ± 0.003
Radius + Ulna	**0.944 ± 0.005**	0.878 ± 0.002
Wrist	0.921 ±0.007	0.875 ± 0.008

Since shape and texture give complementary information, we evaluated the classification performance on feature vectors constructed by concatenating the shape and texture parameters (see Table 4). Comparing the results in Table 3 with Table 4 shows that combining shape and texture parameters achieved better results for the manual annotation than that of texture parameters alone. Although this is expected but it is not always the case for the fully-automated annotation due to noise. For this reason it will be worth investigating, in future work, the effect of combining different classifiers each trained on a different feature type (i.e. Radius shape, Radius texture, Ulna shape, Ulna texture) instead of concatenating features as we did here. Figure 3 shows the full ROC curves for the best results.

Table 4. AUC for Classification using Combined Shape & Texture parameters for manual and fully automated annotation

Shape & Texture	Manual	Fully automated
Radius	0.907 ± 0.008	0.868 ± 0.002
Ulna	0.866 ± 0.013	0.714 ± 0.002
Radius + Ulna	**0.955 ± 0.005**	0.866 ± 0.006
Wrist	0.944 ± 0.003	**0.886 ± 0.009**

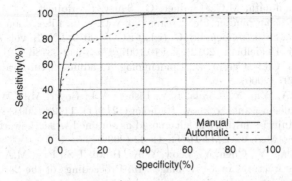

Fig. 3. The ROC curves corresponding to classification achieved by (i) best manual model (i.e. concatenation of shape and texture parameters of Radius and Ulna) and by (ii) best automatic model (i.e. concatenation of shape and texture parameters of Wrist).

5   Conclusions

This paper presents a system that automatically locates the outline of the bones (the radius and ulna), then uses shape and texture features to classify abnormalities. It demonstrates encouraging results. The performance with manual annotation suggests that improving segmentation accuracy will allow significant improvement in classification performance for the automatic system. We are working on expanding our data sets, designing classifiers to focus on specific areas where fractures tend to occur (e.g. the ulnar styloid), and on combining classifiers trained on different types of features instead of concatenating features and train one Random Forest classifier. Our long term goal is to build a system which is reliable enough to help clinicians in A&E to make more reliable decisions.

Acknowledgments. The research leading to these results has received funding from Libyan Ministry of Higher Education and Research. The authors would like to thank Dr. Jonathan Harris, Dr. Matthew Davenport, and Dr. Martin Smith for their collaboration to set up the project, and also thank Jessie Thomson, Luca Minciullo for their useful comments.

References

1. Bayram, F., Çakirolu, M.: DIFFRACT: DIaphyseal Femur FRActure Classifier SysTem. Biocybern. Biomed. Eng. **36**(1), 157–171 (2016)
2. Cao, Y., Wang, H., Moradi, M., Prasanna, P., Syeda-Mahmood, T.F.: Fracture detection in x-ray images through stacked random forests feature fusion. In 2015 IEEE 12th International Symposium on Biomedical Imaging (ISBI), pp. 801–805, April 2015
3. Cootes, T.F., Edwards, G.J., Taylor, C.J.: Active appearance models. IEEE Trans. Pattern Anal. Mach. Intell. **23**(6), 681–685 (2001)
4. Cootes, T.F., Ionita, M.C., Lindner, C., Sauer, P.: Robust and accurate shape model fitting using random forest regression voting. In: Fitzgibbon, A., Lazebnik, S., Perona, P., Sato, Y., Schmid, C. (eds.) ECCV 2012. LNCS, vol. 7578, pp. 278–291. Springer, Heidelberg (2012). doi:10.1007/978-3-642-33786-4_21
5. Court-Brown, C.M., Caesar, B.: Epidemiology of adult fractures: a review. Injury **37**(8), 691–697 (2006)
6. Goldfarb, C.A., Yin, Y., Gilula, L.A., Fisher, A.J., Boyer, M.I.: Wrist fractures: what the clinician wants to know. Radiology **219**(1), 11–28 (2001)
7. Guly, H.R.: Injuries initially misdiagnosed as sprained wrist (beware the sprained wrist). Emerg. Med. J., EMJ **19**(1), 41–42 (2002)
8. Lim, S.E., Xing, Y., Chen, Y., Leow, W.K., Howe, T.S., Png, M.A.: Detection of femur, radius fractures in x-ray images. In: Proceedings of the 2nd International Conference on Advances in Medical Signal and Information Processing, vol. 1, pp. 249–256 (2004)
9. Lindner, C., Thiagarajah, S., Wilkinson, J.M., Consortium, T., Wallis, G.A., Cootes, T.F.: Fully automatic segmentation of the proximal femur using random forest regression voting. Med. Image Anal. **32**(8), 1462–1472 (2013)
10. Lum, V.L.F., Leow, W.K., Chen, Y., Howe, T.S., Png, M.A.: Combining classifiers for bone fracture detection in X-ray images, vol. 1, pp. I-1149–I-1152 (2005)
11. Petinaux, B., Bhat, R., Boniface, K., Aristizabal, J.: Accuracy of radiographic readings in the emergency department. Am. J. Emerg. Med. **29**(1), 18–25 (2011)
12. Porrino, J.A., Maloney, E., Scherer, K., Mulcahy, H., Ha, A.S., Allan, C.: Fracture of the distal radius: epidemiology and premanagement radiographic characterization. AJR, Am. J. Roentgenol. **203**(3), 551–559 (2014)
13. Roberts, M.G., Oh, T., Pacheco, E.M.B., Mohankumar, R., Cootes, T.F., Adams, J.E.: Semi-automatic determination of detailed vertebral shape from lumbar radiographs using active appearance models. Osteoporosis Int. **23**(2), 655–664 (2012)
14. Tian, T.-P., Chen, Y., Leow, W.-K., Hsu, W., Howe, T.S., Png, M.A.: Computing neck-shaft angle of femur for x-ray fracture detection. In: Petkov, N., Westenberg, M.A. (eds.) CAIP 2003. LNCS, vol. 2756, pp. 82–89. Springer, Heidelberg (2003)
15. Wei, C.-J., Tsai, W.-C., Tiu, C.-M., Wu, H.-T., Chiou, H.-J., Chang, C.-Y.: Systematic analysis of missed extremity fractures in emergency radiology. Acta Radiol. **47**(7), 710–717 (2006)
16. Jia, Y., Jiang, Y.: Active contour model with shape constraints for bone fracture detection. In: International Conference on Computer Graphics, Imaging and Visualisation (CGIV 2006), vol. 3, pp. 90–95 (2006)
17. Yap, D.W.H., Chen, Y., Leow, W.K., Howe, T.S., Png, M.A.: Detecting femur fractures by texture analysis of trabeculae. In: Proceedings of the International Conference on Pattern Recognition, vol. 3, pp. 730–733 (2004)

Fast, Intuitive, Vision-Based: Performance Metrics for Visual Registration, Instrument Guidance, and Image Fusion

Ehsan Basafa[✉], Martin Hoßbach, and Philipp J. Stolka

Clear Guide Medical, Baltimore, MD 21211, USA
{basafa,hossbach,stolka}@clearguidemedical.com

Abstract. We characterize the performance of an ultrasound+ computed tomography image fusion and instrument guidance system on phantoms, animals, and patients. The system is based on a visual tracking approach. Using multi-modality markers, registration is unobtrusive, and standard instruments do not require any calibration. A novel deformation estimation algorithm shows externally-induced tissue displacements in real time.

Keywords: Ultrasound · Computed tomography · Image fusion · Instrument guidance · Navigation · Deformable modeling · Computer vision · Metrics

1 Introduction

For many ultrasound (US) operators, the main difficulty in needle-based interventions is keeping hand-held probe, target, and instrument aligned at all times after initial sonographic visualization of the target. In other cases, intended targets are difficult to visualize in ultrasound alone – they may be too deep, occluded, or not echogenic enough. To improve this situation, precise and robust localization of all components – probe, target, needle, and pre- or intra-procedural 3D imaging – in a common reference frame and in real time can help. This allows free motion of both target and probe, while continuously visualizing targets. Easy-to-use image fusion of high resolution 3D imaging such as magnetic resonance (MR) and computed tomography (CT) with real-time ultrasound data is the key next stage in the development of image-guided interventional procedures.

The Clear Guide SCENERGY (Clear Guide Medical, Inc., Baltimore, MD) is a novel CT-US fusion system aiming to provide such user-friendly and accurate guidance. Its main differentiator is the intuitive provision of such fusion and guidance capabilities with only minor workflow changes. The system is cleared through FDA 510(k), CE Mark, and Health Canada license.

2 Image Fusion and Guidance System

The Clear Guide SCENERGY provides CT and US fusion for medical procedures, as well as instrument guidance to help a user reach a target in either modality

© Springer International Publishing AG 2016
R. Shekhar et al. (Eds.): CLIP 2016, LNCS 9958, pp. 9–17, 2016.
DOI: 10.1007/978-3-319-46472-5_2

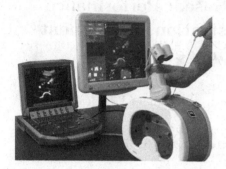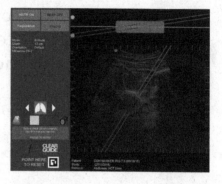

Fig. 1. (a) Clear Guide SCENERGY system, with touchscreen computer, hand-held SuperPROBE (ultrasound probe with mounted Optical Head), connected to a standard ultrasound system. (b) User interface in Fusion Mode, with registered US and CT and overlaid tracked instrument path.

(Fig. 1(a)). Using skin-attached markers (Clear Guide VisiMARKERs) that are visible both optically and radiographically, the system tracks the hand-held US probe pose in real time relative to the patient, and extracts the corresponding CT slice for overlaid display with the current live US slice (Fig. 1(b)). Instrument and target (if selected) are overlaid onto the live CT/US fused view for guidance.

2.1 System

The Optical Head is rigidly attached to standard ultrasound probes via probe-specific brackets, all of which is collectively called the Clear Guide SuperPROBE. Stereo cameras in the Optical Head observe the field of view next to the Super-PROBE, and detect both instruments and markers. Infrared vision and illumination enable this even in low-light environments.

The touchscreen computer provides the user interface and performs all computations. Ultrasound image acquisition and parameterization happens through the user's existing ultrasound and probe system, to which the system is connected through a video connection, capturing frames at full frame rate and resolution. Imaging geometry (depth and US coordinate system) is extracted by real-time pattern matching against known pre-calibrated image modes.

The system receives CT volumes in DICOM format via network from a Picture Archive and Communication System (PACS) or USB mass storage.

3   Interventional Workflow

The clinical workflow (Fig. 2(a)) consists of two functional modes: Registration and Imaging. The system starts in Registration mode (Sect. 3.1) to allow the user to import CT data, and to perform a visual-sweep registration. The operator then switches into Imaging mode (Sect. 3.2), where fused US+CT images and instrument guidance are displayed in real time.

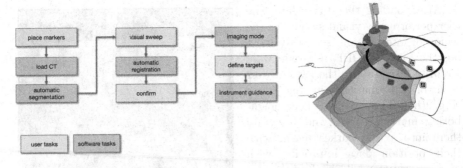

Fig. 2. (a) Workflow for complete image-guided procedure using the SCENERGY system. (b) Example SuperPROBE motion during Visual Sweep Registration showing cameras' fields of view.

3.1 Registration

CT Scan with VisiMARKERs. The registration between pre-procedural CT and the patient relies on multi-modality markers placed on the skin, and their locations' exact reconstruction by the cameras. Thus, it is important to ensure that at least some markers will be visible during the entire procedure. Registration is more robust when marker placement and spacing is irregular and non-symmetric.

In a typical clinical workflow, 5–15 fiducial markers are added to the patient prior to the pre-procedural scan. During loading of that scan, these "early markers" are automatically segmented based on shape and radiopacity. However, the clinician has the option of adding further "late markers" before registration. These provide additional points of reference for later tracking to improve tracking robustness, but do not affect registration. After registration, the system does not differentiate between early and late markers, treating all markers as ground truth for tracking.

The system also segments out the patient skin surface from the CT volume using the Otsu algorithm [5]. This surface is used for three purposes: user reference, aiding in registration, and creating a deformable model (Sect. 3.2).

Visual Tracking. The system continuously scans the stereo camera images for the markers' visual patterns [4] and, through low-level pattern detection, pattern interpretation, stereo reconstruction, and acceptance checking, provides the 6-DoF marker pose estimation for each marker. After registration, the probe pose estimation is based on observations of (subsets of) the markers.

Visual Sweep Registration. "Registration" (the pairing of real-time optical data and the static CT dataset) is performed in two steps: first, visual marker observations are collected to create a 3D marker mesh, and second, image data and observations are automatically matched by searching for the best fit between them. Though this process is not new in itself, the implementation results in a simplification of the user workflow compared to other systems.

After loading the static data, the user performs a "visual sweep" of the region of intervention, smoothly moving the SuperPROBE approximately 15 cm to 20 cm above the patient over each of the markers in big loops (Fig. 2(b)). The sweeps collect neighboring markers' poses and integrate them into a 3D marker mesh, with their position data improving with more observations. The software automatically finds the best correspondence between the observed and segmented markers based on the registration RMS error, normal vector alignment, and closeness to the segmented patient surface. The continuously updated Fiducial Registration Error (FRE) helps in assessing the

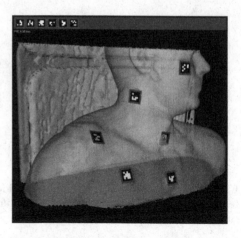

Fig. 3. Visual Sweep registration result, showing markers matched (green) to CT-segmented locations (red). (Color figure online)

associated registration accuracy. Misdetected, shifted, or late markers do not contribute to the FRE or the registration itself, if they fall more than 10 mm from their closest counterpart in the other modality. However, note that the commonly used FRE is not directly correlated to the more clinically relevant Target Registration Error (TRE) [2]. No operator interaction (e.g. manual pairing of segmented and detected markers) is required for automatic registration.

As markers are detected, their relative positions are displayed and mapped onto the segmented patient skin surface according to the best found registration (Fig. 3). This marker mesh is the ground truth for future probe pose estimation.

3.2   Imaging

Fusion Image Guidance. The system constantly reconstructs CT slices from the static volume and overlays them on the US image (Fig. 4) using the current probe pose relative to the observed marker mesh (based on real-time ongoing registration of current observations to the ground truth mesh) and the current US image geometry as interpreted from the incoming real-time US video stream.

Dynamic Targeting. The operator may define a target by tapping on the live US/CT image. Visual tracking allows continuous 3-D localization of the target point relative to the ultrasound probe, fixed in relation to the patient. This "target-lock" mechanism enhances the operator's ability to maintain instrument alignment with a chosen target, independent of the currently visualized slice. During the intervention, guidance to the target is communicated through audio and on-screen visual cues (Fig. 4).

Deformation Modeling. Pressing the ultrasound probe against a patient's body, as is common in most ultrasound-enabled interventions, results in

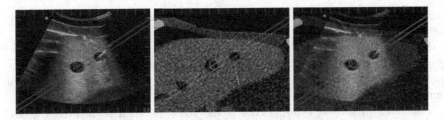

Fig. 4. (a) Live US image, (b) corresponding registered CT slice, (c) fusion image of both modalities (all images showing overlaid instrument and target guidance, with magenta lines indicating PercepTIP [6] needle insertion depth). Note the CT deformation modeling matching the actual US image features. (Color figure online)

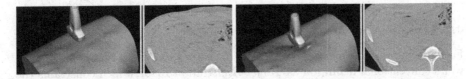

Fig. 5. Surface segmented from CT with tracked probe in-air (a), with probe pressing down on the surface (b).

deformation seen in the real-time ultrasound image. When using image fusion, the static image would then be improperly matched to the ultrasound scan if this effect were not taken into account. Based on probe pose, its geometry, and the patient surface, the system thus estimates collision displacements and simulates the corresponding deformation of the CT slice in real time (Figs. 4 and 5). The underlying non-linear mass-spring-damper model approximates the visco-elastic properties of soft tissues, and is automatically generated and parameterized by the CT's Hounsfield values at the time of loading and segmenting the CT data [1].

4 Performance Metrics

Conventionally, interventional image guidance systems are described in terms of fiducial registration error (FRE, which is simple to compute at intervention time) and target registration error (TRE, which is more relevant, but harder to determine automatically). In addition to that, we also break down the performance evaluation of the presented system into several distinct metrics as follows.

4.1 Segmentation Accuracy and FRE

Distances between hand-selected centers of markers ("gold standard") and those from the automated Clear Guide SCENERGY algorithm indicate segmentation accuracy. Because the automated system considers all voxels of marker-like intensity for centroid computation, we believe the system actually achieves higher precision than manual "ground truth" segmentation which was based on merely selecting the marker corners and finding the center point by 3D averaging.

Segmentation error (automatic segmentation compared to manual center determination) was (0.58 ± 0.4) mm ($n = 2$ pigs, $n = 2$ patients, $n = 5$ phantoms; $n = 64$ markers total, $6 \ldots 11$ markers each), taking approx. 5 s for one complete volume.

Fiducial registration error (FRE) is the RMS between segmented CT and observed camera marker centers. It was (2.31 ± 0.94) mm after visual-sweep registration ($n = 2$ breathing pigs, $n = 7$ breathing patients, $n = 5$ phantoms; $4 \ldots 11$ markers registered for each; all at 0.5 mm CT slice spacing).

No instances of incorrect marker segmentation or misregistration (i.e. resulting wrong matches) were observed (100 % detection rate; $FP = FN = 0$).

4.2 Fusion Accuracy (TRE)

Fusion accuracy was measured as *Tissue Registration Error (TRE)* (in contrast to its conventional definition as *Target Registration Error*, which constrains the discrepancy to just a single target point per registration). It depends on registration quality (marker placement and observations) and internal calibration (camera/US). Fused image pairs (collected by a novice clinical operator; $n = 2$ breathing pigs, $n = 7$ breathing patients, $n = 5$ phantoms) were evaluated to determine fusion accuracy. As tens of thousands of image pairs were collected in every run, we manually selected pairs with good anatomical visualization in both US and CT; however not selecting for good registration, but only for good visibility of anatomical features. To ensure a uniform distribution of selected pairs, we systematically chose one from each block of $m = 350 \ldots 500$ consecutive pairs ($4 \ldots 94$ pairs per run).

Discrepancy lines were manually drawn on each image pair between apparently corresponding salient anatomical features, evenly spaced (approx. 10 lines per pair; $59 \ldots 708$ lines per run) (Fig. 6(a)). After extreme-outlier removal (truncation at $3\times$ interquartile range; those correspond to clearly visible mismatches) and averaging first within (i.e. instantaneous accuracy) and then across pairs per run (i.e. case accuracy) to reduce sampling bias, the resulting *Tissue Registration Error (TRE)* was 3.75 ± 1.63 mm.

4.3 Systematic Error

Systematic error is the cumulative error observed across the entire system, which includes the complete chain of marker segmentation, sweep-based registration, probe tracking, CT slicing, and instrument guidance errors. This performance metric is a "tip-to-tip" distance from the needle point shown in registered ground-truth CT to the same needle point shown by overlaid instrument guidance (Fig. 6(b)). It represents the level of trust one can place in the system if no independent real-time confirmation of instrument poses – such as from US or fluoro – is available. (Note that this metric does not include User Error, i.e. the influence of suboptimal needle placement by the operator.) This metric is sometimes

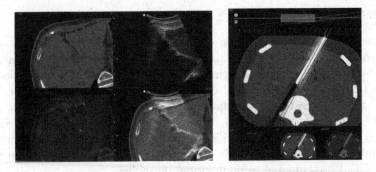

Fig. 6. (a) Tissue Registration Error computation based on discrepancy lines (red). (b) Systematic Error computation based on difference between needle in CT and overlaid instrument guidance. (Color figure online)

referred to as "tracking error" – "the distance between the 'virtual' needle position computed using the tracking data, and the 'gold standard' actual needle position extracted from the confirmation scan" [3]. The total systematic error was found to be (3.99 ± 1.43) mm ($n = 9$ phantoms with FRE (1.23 ± 0.58) mm; with results averaged from $2 \ldots 12$ reachable probe poses per registered phantom). The tracked CT is displayed at $15 \ldots 20$ fps, and instrument guidance at 30 fps.

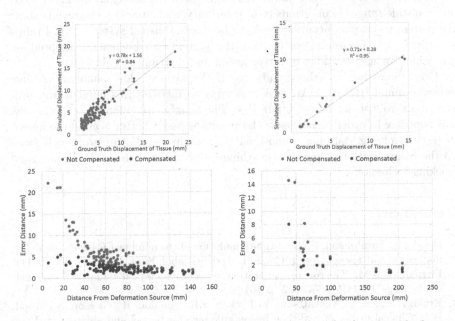

Fig. 7. Deformation simulation results: displacement recovery (top) and residual error (bottom), for ex-vivo liver (left) and in-vivo pig (right)

4.4 Deformation Accuracy

The system simulates deformation of the static CT image to compensate for compression error caused by pressing the probe onto the patient tissue. Performance testing measured the estimated recovery (i.e. simulated displacement for each target divided by original compression displacement) and the residual error (Fig. 7). In a silicone liver dataset [7], recovery was estimated at 78.2 % ($n = 117$ BB targets; $R^2 = 0.84$), whereas an in-vivo porcine dataset yielded 71.4 % ($n = 15$ BB targets; $R^2 = 0.95$) recovery; with the simulation running at 50 fps and a settling time of $1\ldots2$ s. The deformation model thus demonstrates a clear benefit as compared to no deformation model.

5 Conclusion

We described a novel US+CT image fusion and instrument guidance system, based on inside-out visual tracking from hand-held ultrasound probes. It simplifies the user workflow compared to the state of the art, as it provides automatic patient and marker segmentation, allows for rapid "visual sweep" patient/CT registration, works with nearly all standard instruments, and naturally does not suffer from the usual line-of-sight or EM-field-disturbance drawbacks of conventional tracking systems.

A variety of experiments characterized the performance of all workflow steps under a wide range of conditions (lab, veterinary, and clinical). The results show the system to have an accuracy comparable to established systems (e.g. Philips PercuNav [3]). Therefore, we believe, the system can be readily adopted by physicians for user-friendly, intuitive fusion and instrument guidance.

One limitation of this study is the relatively low number of live patient/animal trial runs. Work is underway to increase this number and provide more robust statistical inferences. The number of phantom experiments was kept low in order to not skew the results towards better accuracy inherent in tests involving stationary, non-breathing phantoms. Future work will focus on the compensation of patient-breathing-induced errors using the same visual tracking technology.

References

1. Basafa, E., Farahmand, F.: Real-time simulation of the nonlinear visco-elastic deformations of soft tissues. Int. J. Comput. Assist. Radiol. Surg. **6**(3), 297–307 (2011)
2. Fitzpatrick, J.M.: The role of registration in accurate surgical guidance. Proc. Inst. Mech. Eng. H **224**(5), 607–622 (2010)
3. Krucker, J., Xu, S., Venkatesan, A., Locklin, J.K., Amalou, H., Glossop, N., Wood, B.J.: Clinical utility of real-time fusion guidance for biopsy and ablation. J. Vasc. Interv. Radiol. **22**(4), 515–524 (2011)
4. Olson, E.: AprilTag: a robust and flexible visual fiducial system. In: Proceedings of the IEEE ICRA, pp. 3400–3407 (2011)

5. Otsu, N.: A threshold selection method from gray-level histograms. IEEE Trans. Syst. Man Cybern. **9**(1), 62–66 (1979)
6. Stolka, P.J., Foroughi, P., Rendina, M., Weiss, C.R., Hager, G.D., Boctor, E.M.: Needle guidance using handheld stereo vision and projection for ultrasound-based interventions. In: Golland, P., Hata, N., Barillot, C., Hornegger, J., Howe, R. (eds.) MICCAI 2014, Part II. LNCS, vol. 8674, pp. 684–691. Springer, Heidelberg (2014)
7. Suwelack, S., Röhl, S., Dillmann, R., Wekerle, A.L., Kenngott, H., Müller-Stich, B., Alt, C., Speidel, S.: Quadratic corotated finite elements for real-time soft tissue registration. In: Nielsen, P.M.F., Wittek, A., Miller, K. (eds.) Computational Biomechanics for Medicine: Deformation and Flow, pp. 39–50. Springer, New York (2012)

Stable Anatomical Structure Tracking for Video-Bronchoscopy Navigation

Antonio Esteban-Lansaque[1](✉), Carles Sánchez[1], Agnés Borràs[1],
Marta Diez-Ferrer[2], Antoni Rosell[2], and Debora Gil[1]

[1] Computer Science Department, Computer Vision Center,
UAB, Barcelona, Spain
aesteban@cvc.uab.es
[2] Pneumology Unit, Hospital University Bellvitge,
IDIBELL, CIBERES, Barcelona, Spain

Abstract. Bronchoscopy allows to examine the patient airways for detection of lesions and sampling of tissues without surgery. A main drawback in lung cancer diagnosis is the difficulty to check whether the exploration is following the correct path to the nodule that has to be biopsied. The most extended guidance uses fluoroscopy which implies repeated radiation of clinical staff and patients. Alternatives such as virtual bronchoscopy or electromagnetic navigation are very expensive and not completely robust to blood, mocus or deformations as to be extensively used. We propose a method that extracts and tracks stable lumen regions at different levels of the bronchial tree. The tracked regions are stored in a tree that encodes the anatomical structure of the scene which can be useful to retrieve the path to the lesion that the clinician should follow to do the biopsy. We present a multi-expert validation of our anatomical landmark extraction in 3 intra-operative ultrathin explorations.

Keywords: Lung cancer diagnosis · Video-bronchoscopy · Airway lumen detection · Region tracking

1 Introduction

Lung cancer is one of the most diagnosed cancers among men and women. Actually, lung cancer accounts for 13 % of the total cases with a 5-year global survival rate in patients in the early stages of the disease of 38 % to 67 % and in later stages of 1 % to 8 % [1]. This manifests the importance of detecting and treating lung cancer at early stages, which is a challenge in many countries [2]. Computed tomography (CT) screening programs may significantly reduce the risk of lung cancer death. Diagnostic of solitary peripheral lesions can be diagnosed via bronchoscopy biopsy avoiding complications of other interventions such as

D. Gil—Serra Hunter Fellow

R. Shekhar et al. (Eds.): CLIP 2016, LNCS 9958, pp. 18–26, 2016.
DOI: 10.1007/978-3-319-46472-5_3

transthoracic needle aspiration [3]. However, bronchoscopy navigation is a difficult task in case of solitary peripheral small lesions since according to the Am. Coll. Chest Phys., diagnostic sensitivity of lesions is 78 %, but drops to 34 % for lesions < 2 cm [4]. Actually, to reach a potential lesion bronchoscopists plan the shortest and closest path to the lesion exploring a pre-operative CT scan and, at intervention time, try to reproduce such a path by visual identification of bronchial levels and branch orientation in the bronchoscopy video.

Even for expert bronchoscopists it is difficult to reach a lesion due to the lung's anatomical structure. Images are commonly symmetrical so given a rotated broncoscope the direction to follow is not clearly defined. To assess the navigated path, bronchoscopists use a technique called fluoroscopy to obtain real-time X-ray images of the interior of the lungs. Aside from errors arising from visual interpretation, fluoroscopy implies repeated radiation for, both, clinical staff and patients [5]. In very recent years several technologies (like CT Virtual Bronchoscopy VB or electromagnetic navigation) have been proposed to reduce radiation at intervention time. Virtual Bronchoscopy VB (VB LungPoint or NAVI) is a computer simulation of the video bronchoscope image from CT scans to assess the optimal path to a lesion that, at intervention time, guides the clinician across the planned path using CT-video matching methods. Electromagnetic navigation (inReachTM, SpinDrive) uses additional gadgets which act as a GPS system that tracks the tip of the bronchoscope along the intervention. Although promising, these alternative technologies are not as useful as physicians would like. VB LungPoint and NAVI require manual intra-operative adjustments of the guidance system [6,7], while electromagnetic navigation specific gadgets increase the costs of interventions limiting it use to resourceful entities.

Despite having increased interest in recent years, image processing has not been fully explored in bronchoscopy guiding system. Most of the methods are based on multi-modal registration of CT 3D data to video 2D frames. In [8], shape from shading (SFS) methods are used to extract depth information from images acquired by the bronchoscope to match them to the 3D information given by the CT. One of the disadvantages of such methods is that SFS is very time consuming so it cannot be implemented in real time systems. Other methods try to directly match virtual views of the CT to the current frame of the bronchoscope (2D-3D registration) to find the bronchoscope location [9]. Finally, there are hybrid methods [10] that use a first approximation using epipolar geometry that it is corrected by 2D-3D registration. These 2D-3D registration methods are also very time consuming and can lead to a mismatch in case images are obscured by blood or mucus and bronchi are deformed by patient's coughing.

Anatomical landmarks identified in, both, CT scans and videobronchoscopy frames might be a fast alternative to match the off-line planed path to interventional navigation. Landmark extraction in intra-operative videos is challenging due to the large variety of image artifacts and the unpredicted presence of surgical devices. Recent works [11] have developed efficient video processing methods to extract airways lumen centres that have been used in a matching system [12]. The system codified CT airways using a binary tree and used multiplicity of centres tracked in videos to retrieve the navigation path. In spite of promising results, the method was far from clinical deployment. A main criticism is a too simple matching criteria only based on lumen multiplicity which omitted the airway scene structure and the false positive rate in tracking.

We propose a method that extracts not just lumen centres but also stable lumen regions. Lumen regions are a better strategy for bronchoscopic navigation because they provide more information such as the area of the lumen (proximal, distal) and altogether the hierarchy of the regions. In fact, we represent these regions in a tree that encodes the anatomical structure of bronchoscopic images. Besides, assuming slow motion, we track all the regions using a modified Kalman filter with no velocity and no acceleration that tracks the hierarchy of luminal regions. The capability of intra-operative luminal region tracking is assessed by a multi-expert validation in 3 intra-operative ultrathin explorations.

2   Stable Bronchial Anatomy Tracking

To retrieve bronchial anatomy from videos, lumen regions are extracted using maximally stable extremal regions (MSER) over a likelihood map of lumen center location. These regions are encoded with a hierarchical tree structure that filters regions inconsistent with bronchi anatomy in video frames. Finally, anatomically consistent regions are endowed with temporal continuity across the sequence using a modified Kalman filter.

2.1   Bronchial Anatomy Encoding in Single Frames

The first step to encode the anatomical structure of bronchoscopic images is to find lumen regions candidates. Extraction of lumen regions is based on likelihood maps [11] which indicate the probability of a point to be a lumen centre. In

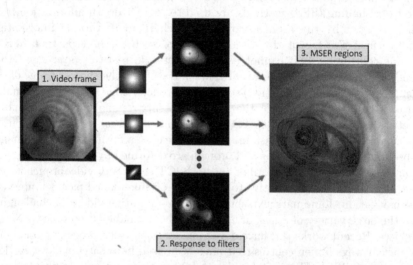

Fig. 1. MSER regions from likelihood maps.

[11], such maps are computed using a single isotropic Gaussian kernel to characterize dark circular areas which under the assumption of central navigation are more probable to be lumen. The use of one single Gaussian kernel limits the extraction of lumen regions to circular regions of the same size which is not fully sensible in interventional videos. To model non-circular lateral bronchi and small distal levels, we compute several likelihood maps using a bank of anisotropic Gaussian filters with different orientations and scales. Gaussian filters have been normalized by their L2 norm to obtain more uniform responses comparable across different scales and degrees of anisotropy. Figure 1 shows the likelihood maps (Fig. 1.2) computed by convolving the left-hand side frame with the bank of Gaussian filters shown in side small images. To suppress outlying small local maxima, likelihood maximal regions are computed using maximally stable extremal regions (MSER) [13]. Finally, all MSER regions are put together (Fig. 1.3) in order to be post-processed in next stages. We note that the collection of MSER regions are a set of elliptical regions following a hierarchy inclusions that should correspond to airways projected from different bronchial levels.

To extract projected airways anatomical structure from MSER regions, we encode their hierarchy using a n-tree using the strategy sketched in Fig. 2. To better illustrate the tree creation we show a synthetic image (Fig. 2.1) that simplifies the image in Fig. 1.3 and a scheme of MSER hierarchy in Fig. 2.2. Since each MSER region should be represented as a node of the tree, we iteratively construct the tree by keeping a list of root and children regions. First, MSER regions are sorted regarding their area in ascending order and the first region of

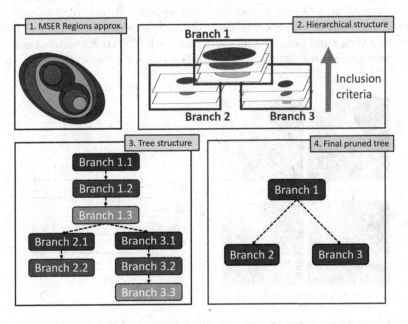

Fig. 2. Tree structure from MSER regions.

the sorted list is added to the root node list and marked as current root. Then, we iteratively consider the next region in the sorted list, add it to the root list and update the children list according to whether the region contains any of the current roots. All roots contained in it are added in the tree structure as child of the node we are examining and are removed from the root list. The tree generated from the hierarchical structure of Fig. 2.2 is shown in Fig. 2.3. Ideally, we would like that each of the bronchial branches that represents a lumen region would correspond to a tree node. This is not the case due to the multiple MSER regions coming from different likelihood maps that lie on a bronchial lumen. Hence, the algorithm also prunes the tree keeping just the highest node of each branch to produce the final tree (Fig. 2.4) encoding bronchial anatomy in images.

2.2   Bronchial Anatomy Tracking Across Sequence Frames

To endow MSER regions with temporal continuity, they are tracked using a modified Kalman filter. For each lumen region at a given frame, a Kalman filter [14] predicts its location in the next frame according to a motion model (constant velocity, constant acceleration) prone to fail in intra-operative videos because lumen movement does not fulfil any of those models. To reduce the impact of sudden variations in motion model, we have implemented a constant position tracker that uses a state vector with zero velocity and zero acceleration. In addition, instead of only using proximity of region centres to match them, we consider their overlap. In this way, our modified tracker matches nearby lumen regions only in case they maintain shape and area so that there is no mismatch in case lumens at different bronchial levels appear. To do so we compute a modified cost matrix with the euclidean distance between the centres of lumen regions at a time i and lumen regions at a time $i+1$. The trick is, when similarity ratio between those regions is small the distance is set to ∞ so that there is no

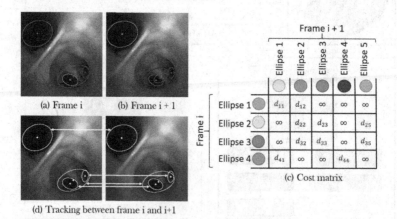

(a) Frame i   (b) Frame i + 1

(d) Tracking between frame i and i+1

(c) Cost matrix

Fig. 3. Region tracking between two consecutive frames and cost matrix. (Color figure online)

matching between those regions. Finally, the Hungarian algorithm [15] is applied
to the cost matrix for optimal matching.

Our tracking of luminal regions is illustrated in Fig. 3. Figure 3a and b show
two frames at time i and $i + 1$ respectively with the luminal regions plotted as
ellipses of different colors. Distances across ellipses at time i and $i + 1$ are given
in the cost matrix shown in Fig. 3c. In those images we can see that there are two
regions which might be mismatched because of its proximity (ellipse 4 at frame
i and ellipse 2 at frame $i + 1$) but their distance is set to ∞ because of its non-
similarity (region overlap). Since our tracker takes into account the position and
the region overlap, it can clearly define the right match. This region matching
allows to track lumens of different bronchi's levels and maintain the anatomical
structure in the image. Finally, in Fig. 3c we can see the regions which have been
correctly matched (white) and those which have not (red).

3   Results

We have compared under intervention conditions the quality of the proposed
tracking according to Sect. 2.2. Method has been applied to 8 sequences extracted
from 3 ultrathin bronchoscopy videos performed for the study of peripheral pulmonary nodules at Hospital de Bellvitge. Videos were acquired using an Olym-
pus Exera III HD Ultrathin videobronchoscope. We have split the 8 sequences
into proximal (up to 6th division) and distal (above 6th) sets to compare also
the impact of the distal level. The maximum bronchial level achieved in our
ultrathin explorations was within 10th and 12th, which is in the range of the
maximum expected level reachable by ultrathin navigation. Sequences contain
bronchoscope collision with the bronchial wall, bubbles due to the anaesthesia
and patient coughing.

For each sequence, we sampled 10 consecutive frames every 50 frames. Such
frames were annotated by 2 clinical experts to set false detections and missed centres. To statistically compare our tracker, ground truth was produced by intersect-
ing the experts' annotations. Ground truth sets were used to compute precision
(Prec) and recall (Rec) for each set of consecutive frames. These scores are taken
for all such sets in distal and proximal fragments for statistical analysis. We have
used a Wilcoxon test data to assess significant differences and confidence intervals,
CI, to report average expected ranges. Table 1 reports CIs for each set of consecutive frames score at proximal, distal and all together (both proximal and distal)
levels. According to these results, it is worth noticing that the proposed method
always has a 100 % of precision and a recall over 84 %. We can see that Recall
at proximal levels is a bit smaller than recall at distal levels. This is due to more
frames with collisions at proximal levels that distort the likelihood model (see Discussion Section). Even so, proximal and distal levels present non-significant differences between them ($p - val > 0.8$ for a Wilcoxon test).

Figure 4 shows regions tracked in consecutive frames selected at distal and
proximal levels. It is worth noticing the capability of our strategy to capture
most distal and lateral bronchi without introducing false positives.

Table 1. Average precision and recall confidence intervals for region tracking.

	Proximal	Distal	Total
Prec	$[1.0, 1.0]$	$[1.0, 1.0]$	$[1.0, 1.0]$
Rec	$[0.84, 0.99]$	$[0.91, 0.98]$	$[0.90, 0.97]$

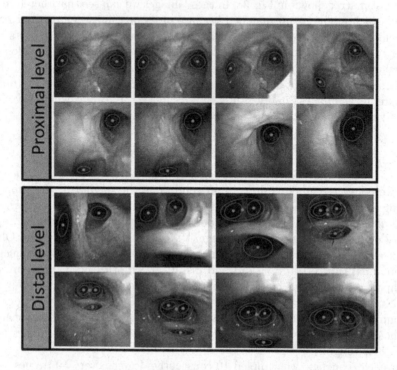

Fig. 4. Frames of tracked regions at proximal and distal levels.

4   Discussion and Conclusions

We have introduced a method that extracts and tracks stable lumen regions at different levels of the bronchial tree. The tracked regions encode the anatomical structure of the scene which can be useful to retrieve the path to the lesion that the clinician should follow to do the biopsy. Results in ultrathin bronchoscopy videos indicate high equal performance of our lumen region tracker based on MSER at proximal and distal levels. Particularly, there are not any false detections (Prec = 1) and the rate of missed lumen regions is under 16 % (Rec > 0.84). Although, non-significant according to a Wilcoxon test, we can appreciate a slight deviation between proximal and distal recall. The reason for such bias is that our model does not satisfy the illumination conditions in carina when collisions happen. This could be solved by making the likelihood maps less restrictive at proximal levels, but does not invalidate our system for bronchoscopic navigation.

Clinicians need guiding systems for distal levels in which we obtain a recall grater than 90 %, at proximal levels, they navigate without any tool just by visually assessing the path.

We conclude that results are promising enough (see the full exploration at https://www.youtube.com/watch?v=CWEHX2KP8YI) to encourage the use of anatomical landmarks in a biopsy guidance system. In Fig. 4 we can see 8 sample images from two videos at distal and proximal level. Images are ordered according to its occurrence in time from left to right and from up to down. As we can see, at proximal levels the anatomical structure of bronchi is easy but at distal levels it becomes more complex. This complex anatomical structure could be used to put in correspondences the anatomical structure extracted from the CT and the anatomical structure extracted from frames recorded by the bronchoscope.

Acknowledgments. This work was supported by Spanish project DPI2015-65286-R, 2014-SGR-1470, Fundació Marató TV3 20133510 and FIS-ETES PI09/90917. Debora Gil is supported by Serra Hunter Fellow.

References

1. Jemal, A., Bray, F., Center, M.M., Ferlay, J., et al.: Global cancer statistics. CA Cancer J. Clin. **61**(2), 69–90 (2011)
2. Reynisson, P.J., Leira, H.O., Hernes, T.N., et al.: Navigated bronchoscopy: a technical review. J. Bronchology Interv. Pulmo. **21**(3), 242–264 (2014)
3. Manhire, A., Charig, M., Clelland, C., Gleeson, F., Miller, R., et al.: Guidelines for radiologically guided lung biopsy. Thorax **58**(11), 920–936 (2003)
4. Donnelly, E.F.: Technical parameters and interpretive issues in screening computed tomography scans for lung cancer. J. Thor. Imag. **27**(4), 224–229 (2012)
5. Shepherd, R.W.: Bronchoscopic pursuit of the peripheral pulmonary lesion: navigational bronchoscopy, radial endobronchial ultrasound, and ultrathin bronchoscopy. Curr. Opin. Pulm. Med. **22**(3), 257–264 (2016)
6. Eberhardt, R., Kahn, N., Gompelmann, D., et al.: Lungpointâa new approach to peripheral lesions. J. Thor. Onco. **5**(10), 1559–1563 (2010)
7. Asano, F., Matsuno, Y., et al.: A virtual bronchoscopic navigation system for pulmonary peripheral lesions. Chest **130**(2), 559–566 (2006)
8. Shen, M., Giannarou, S., Yang, G.-Z.: Robust camera localisation with depth reconstruction for bronchoscopic navigation. IJCARS **10**(6), 801–813 (2015)
9. Rai, L., Helferty, J.P., Higgins, W.E.: Combined video tracking and image-video registration for continuous bronchoscopic guidance. IJCARS **3**(3–4), 315–329 (2008)
10. Luó, X., Feuerstein, M., Deguchi, D., et al.: Development and comparison of new hybrid motion tracking for bronchoscopic navigation. MedIma **16**(3), 577–596 (2012)
11. Sánchez, C., Bernal, J., Gil, D., Sánchez, F.J.: On-line lumen centre detection in gastrointestinal and respiratory endoscopy. In: Erdt, M., Linguraru, M.G., Laura, C.O., Shekhar, R., Wesarg, S., González Ballester, M.A., Drechsler, K. (eds.) CLIP 2013. LNCS, vol. 8361, pp. 31–38. Springer, Heidelberg (2014)

12. Sánchez, C., Diez-Ferrer, M., Bernal, J., Sánchez, F.J., Rosell, A., Gil, D.: Navigation path retrieval from videobronchoscopy using bronchial branches. In: Oyarzun-Laura, C., et al. (eds.) CLIP 2015. LNCS, vol. 9401, pp. 62–70. Springer, Heidelberg (2016). doi:10.1007/978-3-319-31808-0_8
13. Matas, J., Chum, O., Urban, M., Pajdla, T.: Robust wide-baseline stereo from maximally stable extremal regions. Im. Vis. Comp. **22**(10), 761–767 (2004)
14. Haykin, S.S.: Kalman Filtering and Neural Networks. Wiley Online Library, New York (2001)
15. Kuhn, H.W.: The hungarian method for the assignment problem. Naval Res. Logistics Q. **2**(1–2), 83–97 (1955)

Uncertainty Quantification of Cochlear Implant Insertion from CT Images

Thomas Demarcy[1,2]([✉]), Clair Vandersteen[1,3], Charles Raffaelli[4],
Dan Gnansia[2], Nicolas Guevara[3], Nicholas Ayache[1], and Hervé Delingette[1]

[1] Asclepios Research Team, Inria Sophia Antipolis-Mediterranée, Valbonne, France
thomas.demarcy@inria.fr
[2] Department of Cochlear Implant Scientific Research,
Oticon Medical, Vallauris, France
[3] Head and Neck University Institute (IUFC), Nice, France
[4] ENT Imaging Department, Nice University Hospital (CHU), Nice, France

Abstract. Cochlear implants (CI) are used to treat severe hearing loss by surgically inserting an electrode array into the cochlea. Since current electrodes are designed with various insertion depth, ENT surgeons must choose the implant that will maximise the insertion depth without causing any trauma based on preoperative CT images. In this paper, we propose a novel framework for estimating the insertion depth and its uncertainty from segmented CT images based on a new parametric shape model. Our method relies on the posterior probability estimation of the model parameters using stochastic sampling and a careful evaluation of the model complexity compared to CT and μCT images. The results indicate that preoperative CT images can be used by ENT surgeons to safely select patient-specific cochlear implants.

Keywords: Cochlear implant · Uncertainty quantification · Shape modeling

1 Introduction

A cochlear implant (CI) is a surgically implanted device used to treat severe to profound sensorineural hearing loss. The implantation procedure involves drilling through the mastoid to open one of the three cochlear ducts, the scala tympani (ST), and insert an electrode array to directly stimulate the auditory nerve, which induces the sensation of hearing. The post-operative hearing restoration is correlated with the preservation of innervated cochlear structure, such as the modiolus and the osseous spiral lamina, and the viability of hair cells [4].

Therefore for a successful CI insertion, it is crucial that the CI is fully inserted in the ST without traumatizing the neighboring structures. This is a difficult task as deeply inserted electrodes are more likely to stimulate wide cochlear regions but also to damage sensitive internal structures. Current electrode designs include arrays with different lengths, diameters, flexibilities and

© Springer International Publishing AG 2016
R. Shekhar et al. (Eds.): CLIP 2016, LNCS 9958, pp. 27–35, 2016.
DOI: 10.1007/978-3-319-46472-5_4

shapes (straight and preformed). Based on the cochlear morphology selecting the patient-appropriate electrode is a difficult decision for the surgeon [3].

For routine CI surgery, a conventional CT is usually acquired for insertion planning and abnormality diagnosis. However, the anatomical information that can be extracted is limited. Thus, important structures, such as the basilar membrane that separates the ST from other intracochlear cavities, are not visible. On the other hand, high resolution μCT images leads to high quality observation of the cochlear cavities but can only be acquired on cadaveric temporal bones.

Several authors have devised reconstruction methods of the cochlea from CT images by incorporating shape information extracted from μCT images. In particular, Noble et al. [5] and Kjer et al. [2] created statistical shape models of the cochlea based on high-resolution segmented μCT images. Those shape models are created from a small number of μCT images (typically 10) and therefore may not represent well the generality of cochlear shapes that can bias the CT anatomical reconstruction. Baker et al. [1] used a parametric model based on 9 parameters to describe the cochlear as a spiral shell surface. This model was fit to CT images by assuming that the surface model matches high gradient voxels.

In this paper, we aim at estimating to which extent a surgeon can choose a proper CI design for a specific patient based on CT imaging. More specifically, we consider 3 types of implant designs based on their positioning behavior (see Fig. 1f) and evaluate for each design the uncertainty in their maximal insertion depth. If this uncertainty is too large then there is a risk of damaging the ST during the insertion by making a wrong choice. For this uncertainty quantification, we take specific care of the bias-variance tradeoff induced by the choice of the geometric model. Indeed, considering an oversimplified model of the cochlea will typically lead to an underestimation of the uncertainty whereas an overparameterized model would conversely lead to an overestimation of uncertainty.

Therefore, we introduce in this paper a new parametric model of the cochlea and estimate the posterior distribution of its parameters using Markov Chain Monte Carlo (MCMC) method with non informative priors. We devised likelihood functions that relate this parametric shape with the segmentation of 9 pairs of CT and μCT images. The risk of overparameterization is evaluated by measuring the entropy of those posterior probabilities leading to possible correlation between parameters. This generic approach leads to a principled estimation of the probability of CI insertion depths for each of the 9 CT and μCT cases.

2   Methods

2.1   Data

Healthy temporal bones from 9 different cadavers were scanned using CT and μCT scanners. Unlike CT images, which have a voxel size of $0.1875 \times 0.1875 \times 0.25\,\mathrm{mm}^3$ (here resampled to $0.2 \times 0.2 \times 0.2\,\mathrm{mm}^3$) the resolution of μCT images (0.025 mm per voxel) is high enough to identify the basilar membrane that separates the ST from the scala vestibuli (SV) and the scala media. The scala media represents a negligible part of the cochlear anatomy, for simplicity

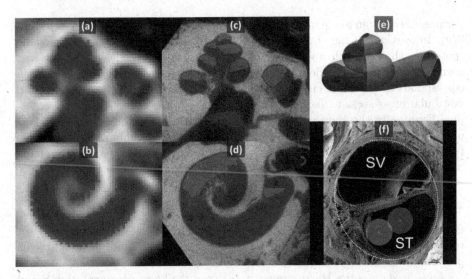

Fig. 1. Slices of CT (a,b) and μCT (c,d) with segmented cochlea (red), ST (blue) and SV (yellow). (e) Parametric model with the ST (blue), the SV (yellow) and the whole cochlea (translucent white). (f) Parametric cross-sections fitted to a microscopic images from [6]. The lateral wall (red), mid-scala (orange) and perimodiolar (yellow) positions of a 0.5 mm diameter electrode are represented. (Color figure online)

purposes, both SV and scala media will be referred as the SV. Since intracochlear anatomy are not visible in CT images, only the cochlea was manually segmented by an head and neck imaging expert, while the ST and the SV were segmented in μCT images (see Fig. 1). All images were rigidly registered using a pyramidal block-matching algorithm and aligned in a cochlear coordinate system [7].

2.2 Parametric Cochlear Shape Model

Since we have a very limited number of high resolution images of the cochlea, we cannot use statistical shape models to represent the generality of those shapes. Instead, we propose a novel parametric model $\mathcal{M}$ of the 3 spiraling surfaces: the whole cochlea, the scala tympani and scala vestibuli (see Fig. 1e). The cochlea corresponds to the surface enclosing the 2 scalae and we introduce a compact parameterization $\mathcal{T} = \{\tau_i\}$ based on 22 parameters for describing the 3 surfaces. This model extends in several ways the ones previously proposed in the literature [1] as to properly capture the complex longitudinal profile of the centerline and the specific shapes of the cross-sections detailed in clinical studies [8]. More precisely, in this novel model, the cochlea and two scalae can be seen as generalized cylinders, i.e. cross-sections swept along a spiral curve. This centerline is parametrized in a cylindrical coordinate system by its radial $r(\theta)$ and longitudinal $z(\theta)$ functions of the angular coordinate θ within a given interval $[0, \theta_f]$. The cross-sections of the ST and SV are modeled by a closed planar curve on which a varying affinity transformation is applied along the centerline, parametrized by an angle of rotation $\alpha(\theta)$ and two scaling parameters $w(\theta)$ and $h(\theta)$. In particular, the three modeled anatomical structures shared the same centerline, the tympanic and vestibular cross-sections are modeled with two half pseudo-cardioids within the same oriented plane while the cochlear cross-section corresponds the minimal circumscribed ellipse of the union of the tympanic and vestibular cross-sections (see Fig. 1f). The center of the ellipse is on the centerline. Eventually the shapes are fully described by 7 one-dimensional functions of θ: $r(\theta)$, $z(\theta)$, $\alpha(\theta)$, $w_{ST}(\theta)$, $w_{SV}(\theta)$, $h_{ST}(\theta)$, $h_{SV}(\theta)$, combinations of simple functions (i.e. polynomial, logarithmic, ...) of θ. The cochlear parametric shape model is detailed in an electronic appendix associated with this paper.

2.3 Parameters Posterior Probability

Given a binary manual segmentation $\mathbf{S}$ of the cochlea from CT imaging, we want to estimate the posterior probability $p(\mathcal{T}|\mathbf{S}) \propto p(\mathbf{S}|\mathcal{T})\,p(\mathcal{T})$ proportional to the product of the likelihood $p(\mathbf{S}|\mathcal{T})$ and the prior $p(\mathcal{T})$.

Likelihood measures the discrepancy between the known segmentation $\mathbf{S}$ and the parametric model $\mathcal{M}(\mathcal{T})$. The shape model can be rasterized, we obtain a binary filled image $\mathcal{R}(\mathcal{T})$ which can be compared to the manual segmentation. Note that the rigid transformation is known after the alignment in cochlear coordinate system [7]. The log-likelihood was chosen to be proportional to the negative square Dice index $s_2(\mathcal{R}(\mathcal{T}), \mathbf{S})$ between the rasterized parametric model and the manually segmented cochlea, $p(\mathbf{S}|\mathcal{T}) \propto \exp(-s_2^2(\mathcal{R}(\mathcal{T}), \mathbf{S})/\sigma^2)$. The square Dice allows to further penalize the shape with low Dice index (e.g. less than 0.7) and σ was set to 0.1 after multiple tests as to provide sufficiently spread posterior distribution.

Prior is chosen to be as uninformative as possible while authorizing an efficient stochastic sampling. We chose an uniform prior for all 22 parameters within a carefully chosen range of values. From 5 manually segmented cochlear shapes from 5 μCT images (different from the 9 considered in this paper), we have extracted the 7 one-dimensional functions of θ modeling the centerline and the cross-sections using a Dijkstra algorithm combined with an active contour estimation. θ was discretized and subsampled 1000 times. The 22 parameters were least-square fit on the subsampled centerline and cochlear points. This has provided us with an histogram of each parameter value from the 5 combined datasets, and eventually the parameter range for the prior was set to the average value plus or minus 3 standard deviations.

Posterior estimation. We use the Metropolis-Hastings Markov Chain Monte-Carlo method for estimating the posterior distribution of the 22 parameters. We choose Gaussian proposal distributions with standard deviations equal to 0.3 % of the whole parameter range used in the prior distribution. Since the parameter range is finite, we use a bounce-back projection whenever the random walk leads a parameter to leave this range.

Posterior from μCT images. In μCT images, the scala tympani and vestibuli can be segmented separately as $\mathbf{S}_{ST}$ and $\mathbf{S}_{SV}$ thus requiring a different likelihood function. The 2 scalae generated by the model $\mathcal{M}(\mathcal{T})$ are separately rasterized as $\mathcal{R}_{ST}(\mathcal{T})$ and $\mathcal{R}_{SV}(\mathcal{T})$ and compared to the 2 manual segmentations using a single multi-structure Dice index $s_3(\mathcal{R}_{ST}(\mathcal{T}), \mathcal{R}_{SV}(\mathcal{T}), \mathbf{S}_{ST}, \mathbf{S}_{SV})$. This index is computed as the weighted average of the 2 Dice indices associated with the 2 scalae. The likelihood function is then $p(\mathbf{S}_{ST}, \mathbf{S}_{SV} | \mathcal{T}) \propto \exp(-s_3^2/\sigma^2)$.

2.4   Controlling Model Complexity

We want to limit the extent of overestimation of uncertainty induced by our rich parametric model. Therefore, we look at the observability of each parameter through its marginalized posterior distribution $p(\tau_i | \mathbf{S}) = \int \int_{\tau_j \neq \tau_i} p(\mathcal{T} | \mathbf{S})\, d\tau_j$. In an ideal scenario, all model parameters should be observable thus indicating that we have not overparameterized the cochlear shape. Therefore we consider the *information gain* $\mathcal{IG}(\tau_i) = -\int_{\tau_i} p(\tau_i) \log p(\tau_i)\, d\tau_i + \int_{\tau_i} p(\tau_i | \mathbf{S}) \log p(\tau_i | \mathbf{S})\, d\tau_i$ computed as difference of entropy between the prior (uniform) distribution and the marginal posterior distribution. The entropy is estimated by binning the distributions using 256 bins covering the range defined by the uniform prior. A low information gain indicates either that the parameter has no observed influence on the shape or that it is correlated with another set of parameters such that many combinations of them lead to the same shape. To test if we are in the former situation, we simply check if the parameter i decreases significantly the likelihood around the maximum *a posteriori* (MAP) by plotting the probability $p(\tau_i | \mathbf{S}, \mathcal{T}_{-i}^{\mathrm{MAP}})$.

2.5   Clinical Metrics

We consider three types of electrodes having the same constant diameter of 0.5 mm. Straight electrodes follow the lateral (outer) wall of the ST, whereas perimodiolar ones follow the modiolar (inner) wall of the ST and mid-scala electrodes are located in the geometric center of the cross-section (see Fig. 1f).

For a given parameter $\mathcal{T}$ and a certain type of electrode, it is relatively simple to compute its trajectory in the ST, by considering each cross-section of the parametric shape model and positioning the center of the CI relative to the inner and outer wall. Furthermore, the maximum insertion depth of a CI $l^{Max}(\mathcal{T})$ can be computed by the arc length of the curve defined by the locus of the electrode positions and by testing if the inscribed circle of the ST boundaries is larger than the electrode. We propose to estimate the posterior probability $p(l^{Max} | \mathbf{S})$ for each CI type by marginalizing over the set of cochlea parameters: $p(l^{Max} | \mathbf{S}) = \int_{\mathcal{T}} p(\mathcal{T} | \mathbf{S})\, l^{Max}(\mathcal{T})\, d\mathcal{T}$. Similarly, we can compute the prior probability of insertion depth which is governed by the prior of the set of parameters: $p(l^{Max}(\mathcal{T})) = \int_{\tau_i} p(\mathcal{T}) l^{Max}(\mathcal{T})\, d\tau_i$.

3   Results

3.1   Model Complexity Evaluation

For each image, 20,000 iterations of the MCMC estimation were performed using a 3.6 GHz Intel Xeon processor machine. The computational time per iteration is less than 4 s for the CT images and less than 20 s for the μCT images. The MCMC mean acceptance rate is 0.38.

The Dice index between the samples corresponding to the maximum *a posteriori* probability (MAP) and the manual segmentations are summarized in Fig. 2(a). Note that s_3 indices are lower on μCT because it considers more substructures (ST and SV) than s_2 indices on CT (cochlea only). A careful inspection of the two structures in Fig. 2b,c suggests that our parametric model has enough degree of freedom to account the complexity of the cochlear shape. The model even appears to regularize the incomplete manual segmentation without overfitting the noise. The mean surface error between the segmented μCT images and the maximum a posteriori models estimated from segmented CT images is less than 0.3 mm. This error depends on the complexity of the model, the rigid registration and the segmentations (independently performed for each modality) but still comparable with the score of 0.2 mm obtained with statistical shape models for cochlear substructures segmentations in CT [5].

On μCT scans, 78 % of the cross-sections parameters have an *information gain* greater than 0.1, while the mean information gain over the 22 parameters is $\overline{IG} = 0.41$. Furthermore, we checked that on μCT scans, for all parameters, any local variation leads to a significant decrease of likelihood $p(\tau_i|\mathbf{S}, \mathcal{T}_{-i}^{MAP})$ and thus showing an influence on the observed shape. This implies that some parameters might be correlated and that shapes may be described by different parameters combinations. Thus we may slightly overestimate the uncertainty (and minimize bias) which is preferable than underestimating it through an oversimplified model. Setting some of those parameters to a constant may be a too strong assumption given that only 9 patient data are considered and therefore we decided to keep the current set of 22 parameters.

On CT scans, 28 % of the cross-sections parameters have an *information gain* greater than 0.1 and $\overline{IG} = 0.23$. The information gain is smaller for CT images than μCT images, which is expected as far less details are visible. In particular, the two scalae are not distinguishable making their model parameters unidentifiable.

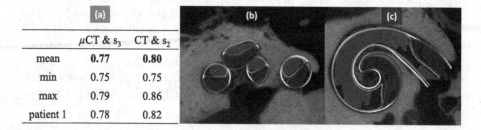

	(a)	
	μCT & s_3	CT & s_2
mean	**0.77**	**0.80**
min	0.75	0.75
max	0.79	0.86
patient 1	0.78	0.82

Fig. 2. (a) Dice indices between the MAP and manual segmentation. (b) and (c) Shape models of the cochlea (light line) of the MAP of patient 1 with the segmented ST (blue) and SV (orange) on μCT images. (Color figure online)

3.2   CT Uncertainty Evaluation

We evaluate the posterior probability of the maximal insertion depth $p(l^{Max}|\mathbf{S})$ for each patient, modality and electrode design. Their cumulative distribution function (CDF) can be clinically interpreted, as it expresses the probability that the maximal insertion depth of a cochlea is less or equal than a given value. Therefore if an electrode has a length l, it also indicates the probability to traumatize the cochlea (if fully inserted). Hence maximal insertion depth corresponding to a CDF of 5 %, can be understood as a 95 % chance that the electrode actually fits in the ST. The CDF accounts for the uncertainty in the whole shape, including cochlear length or diameter. A cochlea with a longer or larger ST would naturally result in a CDF shifted to the right.

The mean standard deviation of the distributions across the patients and electrode designs (see Table 1) shows that uncertainty with CT images is greater than μCT images but still more informative than the prior. To evaluate the bias of maximal insertion depth estimated from CT images we measure the mean discrepancy between the estimation from μCT and CT images. Figure 3b shows the estimation differences between modalities for the worse case, namely straight electrodes. We must stress that all maximal insertion depths are underestimated

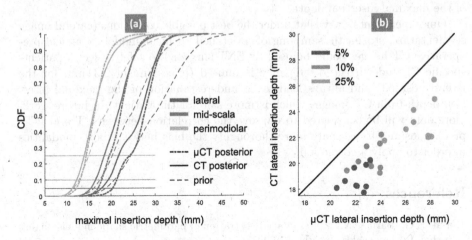

Fig. 3. (a) CDF of the maximal insertion depth estimation for Patient 1. (b) Maximal insertion depth estimation discrepancy between CT and μCT for electrodes following lateral wall at different quantiles (5 %, 10 % and 25 %). Note that the lateral position is the least favorable result in terms of discrepancy between modalities (see Table 1).

Table 1. Statistics summaries of CDF of the maximum insertion depth for all patients and electrode designs (including standard deviation and average discrepancy)

Standard deviation (mm)			Discrepancy between CT and μCT (mm)		
μCT posterior	CT posterior	prior	lateral	mid-scala	perimodiolar
3.42	4.14	5.54	2.34	1.32	0.92

with CT images. The ST is usually larger than the SV at the first basal turn [8] and this information is not explicitly embedded in the prior. Since only little cross-section information can be inferred from CT images, we could hypothesize that the diameters of the ST are more likely to be underestimated with CT images, leading to underestimate insertion depth.

4   Conclusion

In this study, we have proposed a novel parametric model for detailed cochlea shape reconstruction. We evaluated its complexity in order to optimize the uncertainty quantification of intracochlear shapes from CT images. Based on anatomical considerations, our results introduce a measurements of the risk of trauma given a cochlear design and an insertion depth. Most of the CI have a linear electrode depth between 10 and 30 mm, corresponding to the range within which our results are the most revealing. For this data set, the maximal insertion depth spans a 4 mm range. One cochlea (Patient 4) presents a deeper maximal insertion depth than others, we observed that it had a high number of cochlear turns (3.08 compared to an average of 2.6) which was confirmed by a radiologist on μCT. This exemplifies the importance of providing a patient-specific estimation of the maximal insertion depth.

Our experiments show that under the best possible conditions (careful image segmentation, stochastic sampling of a detailed cochlear model), classical preoperative CT images could be used by ENT surgeons to safely select a patient-specific CI. Indeed, the discrepancy is limited (maximum of 2.34 mm for the lateral position) and always lead to an underestimation of the maximal insertion depth from CT images which is more safe for the patient. In future work, more data will be considered to improve the correlation between CT and μCT predictions and to estimate more thoroughly the bias between both modalities in order to apply a correction.

References

1. Baker, G., Barnes, N.: Model-image registration of parametric shape models: fitting a shell to the cochlea. Insight J. (2005)
2. Kjer, H.M.: Modelling of the Human Inner Ear Anatomy and Variability for Cochlear Implant Applications. Ph.D. thesis (2015)
3. van der Marel, K.S., et al.: Diversity in cochlear morphology and its influence on cochlear implant electrode position. Ear Hear. **35**(1), e9–e20 (2014)
4. Nadol, J.B.: Patterns of neural degeneration in the human cochlea and auditory nerve: implications for cochlear implantation. Otolaryngol. Head Neck Surg. **117**(3), 220–228 (1997)
5. Noble, J.H., et al.: Automatic segmentation of intracochlear anatomy in conventional CT. IEEE Trans. Biomed. Eng. **58**(9), 2625–32 (2011)
6. Rask-Andersen, H., et al.: Human cochlea: anatomical characteristics and their relevance for cochlear implantation. Anat. Rec. **295**(11), 1791–811 (2012)

7. Verbist, B.M., et al.: Consensus panel on a cochlear coordinate system applicable in histologic, physiologic, and radiologic studies of the human cochlea. Otol. Neurotol. **31**(5), 722–30 (2010)
8. Wysocki, J.: Dimensions of the human vestibular and tympanic scalae. Hear. Res. **135**(1–2), 39–46 (1999)

Validation of an Improved Patient-Specific Mold Design for Registration of In-vivo MRI and Histology of the Prostate

An Elen[1]([✉]), Sofie Isebaert[1], Frederik De Keyzer[2], Uwe Himmelreich[3], Steven Joniau[4], Lorenzo Tosco[4], Wouter Everaerts[4], Tom Dresselaers[3], Evelyne Lerut[3], Raymond Oyen[2,3], Roger Bourne[5], Frederik Maes[6], and Karin Haustermans[1]

[1] Laboratory of Experimental Radiotherapy,
Department of Oncology, KU Leuven, Leuven, Belgium
an.elen@kuleuven.be
[2] Department of Radiology, University Hospitals Leuven, Leuven, Belgium
[3] Department of Imaging and Pathology,
University Hospitals Leuven, Leuven, Belgium
[4] Department of Urology, University Hospitals, Leuven, Belgium
[5] Discipline of Medical Radiation Sciences, University of Sydney, Sydney, Australia
[6] Department of Electrical Engineering (ESAT/PSI), KU Leuven, Leuven, Belgium

Abstract. Fusion of in-vivo magnetic resonance imaging (MRI) with whole mount histology of the prostate is facilitated by the use of a patient-specific mold, that is designed from in-vivo MRI. The mold defines specific sectioning planes with the same orientation and position relative to the prostate as the stack of MRI slices, reducing the registration problem from a 3D to a 2D problem. We present an innovative mold design that specifies the in- and outflow of the urethra as additional landmarks for correct positioning of the prostate in the mold, that allows for the fresh prostate tissue to be fixated inside the mold such that its in-vivo shape is maintained, and that allows for ex-vivo MRI of the prostate in the mold in alignment with in-vivo MRI using the mold as reference frame. Using high-resolution 3D ex-vivo MRI aligned with in-vivo MRI, we demonstrate that our improved mold design results in a more accurate positioning of the prostate inside the mold, significantly reducing out-of-plane rotational offsets. Initial results show that the proposed workflow has the potential to provide detailed histopathological ground truth for the quantitative interpretation of in-vivo and ex-vivo MRI in prostate cancer.

1 Introduction

Radiation therapy treatment of prostate cancer is evolving towards focal boosting strategies, to maximize both tumor control and normal tissue sparing. To this end, accurate identification of the exact location and boundaries of the tumor are of utmost importance, but so far, there is no consensus on the ideal MRI

© Springer International Publishing AG 2016
R. Shekhar et al. (Eds.): CLIP 2016, LNCS 9958, pp. 36–43, 2016.
DOI: 10.1007/978-3-319-46472-5_5

sequence to do so. Validation against gold standard whole mount pathology is therefore necessary, but this is not trivial. Several approaches for comparing imaging results with histological findings have been used in literature, going from lesion- or sector-based analyses [1–3] over visual comparison or direct registration of the 3D MRI volume with the 2D histological slices [4]. Histology to in-vivo MRI registration is a complicated problem due to the typically low out-of-plane resolution of both sets of images, possible deformation of the histology slices and the limited amount of detail in the in-vivo MRI images, which makes it hard to find corresponding tissue points in both images. Reconstruction of the histology slices into a 3D stack makes the registration problem of histology to in-vivo MRI a 3D problem [5,6]. However, due to the low out-of-plane resolution and resulting sparse 3D data, the registration problem is usually reduced to a set of 2D problems, by visually [7,8] or automatically [9] selecting the most corresponding MRI slice for every histology image. Of course, this is only valid if the orientation of the MRI planes is identical to that of the histological sections. To ensure this, several prostate sectioning devices have been developed. Some require visual orientation and unconstrained positioning of the prostate in the device [7,10]. Others use a mold with a patient-specific prostate shaped cavity to position the sectioning planes relative to the prostate [11,12]. This would result in precisely corresponding 2D histology and MRI slices, provided that the prostate specimen is correctly positioned inside the mold. Using an innovative mold design that enables high-resolution, high-field strength 3D ex-vivo MRI of the prostate tissue inside the mold, we show that this is not guaranteed and that significant out-of-plane rotational offsets may occur despite the use of the mold. The presented improved mold design uses additional landmarks to prevent such mispositioning. Ex-vivo MRI is not only valuable for validation purposes, but also simplifies the histology to in-vivo MRI registration workflow.

2   Registration Workflow and Improved Mold Design

Figure 1 shows an overview of the workflow to register histology to in-vivo MRI, in order to obtain a gold standard for tumor localization and delineation in in-vivo MRI, using high-resolution ex-vivo MRI as intermediate reference to facilitate the registration.

An in-vivo T2-weighted MRI image stack is acquired with similar orientation and slice spacing as preferred for histological sectioning, in our case typically para-axial orthogonal to the urethra outflow. (Para-) sagittal and coronal T2-weighted image stacks are acquired as well and the prostate is manually delineated in all 3 stacks simultaneously, by visualizing the intersection of each contour drawn in any image slice with all slices in the other stacks, such that a consistent 3D delineation is obtained from which the prostate shape is reconstructed. Next, a mold template, consisting of left and right halves, with predefined parallel cutting slots is positioned around the prostate shape such that the cutting slots exactly coincide with the imaging planes. A patient-specific mold is obtained by subtracting the prostate shape from the mold template, and is then 3D printed.

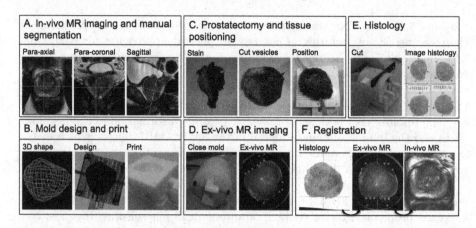

Fig. 1. Overview of the entire workflow. In-vivo MRI images are manually segmented to design a patient-specific mold, in which the prostate tissue is positioned after prostatectomy. Ex-vivo MRI is acquired of the prostate while in the mold, before cutting the tissue and acquiring histology images. The ex-vivo MRI stack is used as high-detail intermediate image to facilitate the histology to in-vivo MRI registration.

We present an improved mold design with the following main and unique features as illustrated in Fig. 2:

1. The position and direction of the in- and outflow of the urethra at the prostate surface are indicated in the in-vivo MRI images and are replicated in the mold as tube shaped openings. These are used as guides for a urethra catheter when positioning the prostate in the mold.
2. Infiltration holes are added to the mold, allowing the tissue to be fixated while in the mold. By placing the prostate in the mold prior to fixation, it is fixated in its in-vivo shape, minimizing possible deformation of the tissue [13] and minimizing positioning difficulties due to tissue fixation-induced rigidity [11].
3. The overall shape and size of the mold are adjusted to fit exactly in the bore of a high-field strength (9.4T) preclinical MRI scanner with 72 mm inside diameter, while contained in a Plexiglas container tube filled with formalin. Hence, high-resolution ex-vivo MRI can be obtained of the prostate in the mold. Several landmarks that are fluid filled when the mold is immersed, are visible during ex-vivo scanning and enable the positioning of the ex-vivo MRI planes in correspondence with the in-vivo MRI planes.

After prostatectomy, the prostate is stained such that the right and left half can be distinguished, the seminal vesicles are removed and a catheter is inserted through the urethra. The prostate is then positioned in the mold guided by the catheter holes. After closing the mold with straps, the catheter is removed and the tissue is fixated overnight using formalin, while in the mold. The mold is then placed in a tubular container filled with formalin and imaged with high-field ex-vivo MRI, to obtain high-detail images. A stack of T2-weighted images

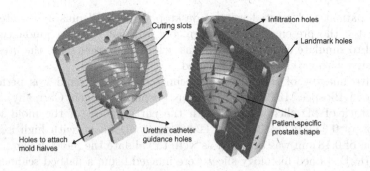

Fig. 2. Proposed patient-specific prostate mold design with indication of the main features.

is acquired at the location of the cutting slots of the mold, thus corresponding to the in-vivo MRI slices.

After ex-vivo imaging, the prostate specimen is sliced inside the mold using the cutting slots and processed using the standard pathological workup. The thick sections are embedded in paraffin and thin sections are sliced from these macro blocks using a microtome. The thin sections are then hematoxylin-eosin (H&E) stained and imaged using a flatbed scanner.

The registration of the stained histology slices to in-vivo MRI is then addressed in two steps, using ex-vivo MRI as intermediate reference. First, the in- and ex-vivo MRI images are rigidly registered, assuming possible ex-vivo shrinking of the tissue to be negligible at this stage [11] and geometric distortion of the ex-vivo MRI images to be limited. As the mold was created from in-vivo MRI delineations, it can be directly overlaid on the in-vivo MRI image, reducing the ex- to in-vivo MRI registration to the simple matching of the mold shape in both image stacks. Secondly, a slice-by-slice 2D non-rigid registration is performed to align the histology and ex-vivo MRI image slices, guided by the many tissue features that are visible in both high-detail images. The Elastix registration package [14] is used for all registrations.

3   Validation of Mold Design

3.1   Image Acquisition

This study was approved by the local Institutional Review Board and written informed consent was obtained from all patients. Six patients with biopsy proven prostate cancer who were scheduled for robotic assisted laparoscopic prostatectomy were included in this study. They all had Gleason score 6 or 7 and different clinical T-stages.

In-vivo imaging was performed on a 1.5 T (Siemens SonataVision, Patients 1–3) or 3T (Philips Ingenia, Patients 4–6) MRI unit. The prostate was delineated by an experienced radiologist in 3 orthogonal T2-weighted in-vivo MRI stacks with a resolution of $0.47 \times 0.47 \times 3$ mm and a patient-specific mold was designed for each patient and printed using a desktop PP3D UP! plus 3D printer. For Patients 1–3 the presented mold design, but without catheter guidance holes was used to simulate classic mold designs, while for Patients 4–6 the presented mold design with catheter holes was used.

Ex-vivo imaging of the prostate specimen inside the mold was performed using a 9.4T Biospec MRI scanner (Bruker Biospin, Ettlingen, Germany). Apart from a stack of 2D slices aligned with the cutting slots of the mold with a resolution of $0.25 \times 0.25 \times 3$ mm, a T2-weighted 3D image with high isotropic resolution of 0.18 mm was acquired as well, to validate the mold design.

The H&E stained histology slices were imaged using a flatbed scanner with a resolution of 0.042×0.042 mm.

3.2 Evaluation

The correspondence between in-vivo MRI and histology is based on the assumption that the prostate specimen is correctly positioned in the mold. To evaluate the validity of this assumption, we manually indicated corresponding tissue landmarks in the 3D ex-vivo MRI image and in-vivo MRI image stacks. Both image sets were rigidly aligned solely based on the mold itself and the same transformation was applied to the landmarks. The residual misalignment between them after mold-based registration was visually assessed and quantified by the rigid transformation T_r. The rotation angles derived from T_r, i.e. the angular offsets between the in-vivo situation and the position of the prostate specimen inside the mold, which ideally should be zero, are summarized in Table 1.

For all 3 cases for which a mold without catheter guides was used (Patients 1–3), significant out-of-plane rotations up to almost 35° were found, especially around the left/right axis. For a slice spacing of 3 mm and a typical prostate extent of 4 cm, a mispositioning of the specimen by 8° around the center already results in tissue displacements of 1 slice. Figure 3 shows the mold-based alignment of the 3D ex-vivo MRI with the 3 orthogonal in-vivo MRI stacks of Patient

Table 1. Residual rotational offsets [in degrees] around each axis for mold-based registration between in-vivo and ex-vivo MRI as determined using internal tissue landmarks, for 3 cases without and 3 cases with catheter guidance embedded in the mold.

	Prostate volume [cc]	Catheter guides	Left-right (out-of-plane)	Antero-posterior (out-of-plane)	Cranio-caudal (in-plane)
Patient 1	50.1	No	12.3	−6.2	3.9
Patient 2	31.2	No	34.6	0.7	7.4
Patient 3	24.6	No	12.2	−0.4	−2.4
Patient 4	56.6	Yes	2.0	−2.2	−10.4
Patient 5	47.8	Yes	1.6	−1.2	1.9
Patient 6	49.3	Yes	−1.6	2.7	1.2

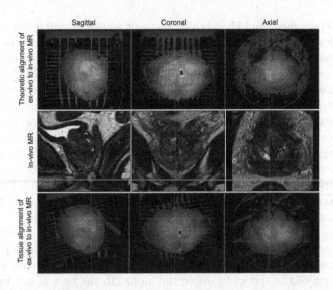

Fig. 3. Alignment of the 3 orthogonal in-vivo MRI stacks (middle row) of Patient 1 to the 3D ex-vivo image of the prostate specimen solely based on the mold (top row) and on internal tissue landmarks (bottom row), illustrating significant residual rotational misalignment for mold-based registration.

1, as well as their corrected landmark-based alignment, illustrating the rotational mispositioning of the specimen in the mold.

For all 3 cases for which a mold with catheter guides was used (Patients 4–6), out-of-plane rotations were smaller than 3°, resulting in maximal tissue displacements of less than half a slice. For Patient 4, an in-plane rotational offset of around 10° was found. For Patients 5 and 6, care was taken to position the cutting plane of the seminal vesicles symmetrical in both mold halves to prevent in-plane rotation.

This quantifies the ex- to in-vivo MRI registration. To validate the second part of the registration workflow, non-rigidly registering histology to ex-vivo MRI, we manually indicated corresponding landmarks in every high-detail histology and ex-vivo MRI slice. The histology landmarks were transformed to the ex-vivo MRI using the found transformation field and the mean distance between both sets of landmarks was calculated to be 0.90 ± 0.56 and 0.94 ± 0.44 mm for Patients 5 and 6 respectively (the correctly positioned specimens).

4   Discussion and Conclusion

We presented an innovative mold design to support the pathological workup of the prostate without altering it and to facilitate the subsequent registration of the histological slices to in-vivo MRI. The unique features of our design include infiltration holes allowing fixation of the fresh tissue in the mold to retain its in-vivo shape, a cylindrical outer shape that fits inside the bore of a high-field strength MRI scanner, liquid filled channels to provide MR-visible landmarks and catheter holes to provide extra guidance for more accurate specimen positioning. This improved mold design offers the possibility to scan the prostate inside the mold, after or prior to fixation, using high resolution ex-vivo MRI, such that corresponding in-vivo MRI, ex-vivo MRI and histology slices are obtained with the same orientation and position relative to the prostate specimen. This opens many opportunities for addressing a variety of research questions.

First, ex-vivo MRI can be used as intermediate reference for histology to in-vivo MRI registration. The high-detail ex-vivo MRI images are easily registered to the in-vivo MRI images based on the mold and provide a rich set of features to guide the non-rigid registration of the histology slices with ex-vivo MRI slices. As a proof-of-concept, the accuracy of histology to ex-vivo MRI and ex- to in-vivo MRI registration was quantified for 2 patients.

Secondly, the possibility to scan the prostate inside the mold with high 3D resolution and contrast allows to validate the underlying assumption of mold-based registration that the patient-specific shape of the mold uniquely constrains the positioning of the specimen inside the mold. To the best of our knowledge, this has not yet been validated despite the frequent use of such molds.

Based on the alignment of internal tissue landmarks as visible in 3D ex-vivo MRI on the one hand and multi-planar in-vivo MRI stacks on the other hand, we showed that the traditional mold design may still result in significant rotational inaccuracies in the positioning of the tissue. This may be attributed to various factors that all introduce some residual degrees of freedom when positioning the specimen inside the mold. First of all, the prostate shape is rather simple and somewhat cylindrically symmetric with little local features. Secondly, the shape of the mold may deviate from that of the excised prostate specimen due to uncertainties in the delineation and during the prostatectomy itself, such that both may not be perfectly fitting. Thirdly, as the tissue is placed inside the mold prior to fixation, it is slightly deformable.

We showed that these residual degrees of freedom could be substantially reduced by extending the mold with catheter guides at the location and with the orientation of the urethra in- and outflow of the prostate. By inserting a catheter through the urethra, the positioning of the specimen inside the mold is further restricted by its in- and outflow location on the prostate surface. By additionally taking care that the plane, along which the seminal vesicles were cut, is placed symmetrically in both mold halves, precise positioning of the tissue in the mold is achieved with residual rotational inaccuracies smaller than $3°$.

More accurate positioning of the specimen inside the mold and the availability of high resolution ex-vivo MRI both contribute to improving the registration accuracy between histology and in-vivo MRI. In the end, this will help to evaluate the potential of different in-vivo and ex-vivo MRI techniques for tumor detection and delineation and to correlate quantitative image features with the underlying (patho-)physiology based on ground truth as provided by histopathology. This will improve the predictive value of MRI and our understanding of its current limitations. Vice versa, the fusion with in-vivo and ex-vivo MRI could be used by pathologists to guide the quick assessment of suspect tissue regions.

References

1. Haider, M.A., van der Kwast, T.H., Tanguay, J., Evans, A.J., Hashmi, A.T., Lockwood, G., Trachtenberg, J.: Combined T2-weighted and diffusion-weighted MRI for localization of prostate cancer. AJR **189**, 323–328 (2007)
2. Turkbey, B., Pinto, P.A., Mani, H., Bernardo, M., Pang, Y., McKinney, Y.L., Khurana, K., Ravizzini, G.C., Albert, P.S., Merino, M.J., Choyke, P.L.: Prostate cancer: value of multiparametric MR imaging at 3T for detection - histopathologic correlation. Radiology **255**, 89–99 (2010)
3. Isebaert, S., Van den Bergh, L., Haustermans, K., Joniau, S., Lerut, E., De Wever, L., De Keyzer, F., Budiharto, T., Slagmolen, P., Van Poppel, H., Oyen, R.: Multiparametric MRI for prostate cancer localization in correlation to whole-mount histopathology. JMRI **37**, 1392–1401 (2013)
4. Meyer, C., Ma, B., Kunju, L.P., Davenport, M., Piert, M.: Challenges in accurate registration of 3-D medical imaging and histopathology in primary prostate cancer. Eur. J. Nucl. Med. Mol. Imaging **40**(Suppl. 1), S72–S78 (2013)
5. Bart, S., Mozer, P., Hemar, P., Lenaour, G., Comperat, E., Renard-Penna, R., Chartier-Kastler, E., Troccaz, J.: MRI-histology registration in prostate cancer. In: Surgetica 2005, Merloz P., Troccaz J. (ed.) Sauramps Medical, pp. 361–367 (2005)
6. Orczyk, C., Mikheev, A., Rosenbrantz, A.B., Melamed, J., Taneja, S.S., Rusinek, H.: Imaging of prostate cancer: a platform for 3D co-registration of in-vivo MRI ex-vivo MRI and pathology. Proc. SPIE Int. Soc. Opt. Eng. **8316** (2012)
7. Kalavagunta, C., Zhou, X., Schmechel, S.C., Metzger, G.J.: Registration of in vivo prostate MRI and pseudo-whole mount histology using local affine transformations guided by internal structures (LATIS). JMRI **41**, 1104–1114 (2015)
8. Chappelow, J., Bloch, B.N., Rofsky, N., Genega, E., Lenkinski, R., DeWolf, W., Madabhushi, A.: Elastic registration of multimodal prostate MRI and histology via multiattribute combined mutual information. Med. Phys. **38**(4), 2005–2018 (2011)
9. Xiao, G., Bloch, B.N., Chappelow, J., Genega, E.M., Rofsky, N.M., Lenkinski, R.E., Tomaszewski, J., Feldman, M.D., Rosen, M., Madabhushi, A.: Determining histology-MRI slice correspondences for defining MRI-based disease signatures of prostate cancer. Comput. Med. Imag. Grap. **35**, 568–578 (2011)
10. Hong Chen, L., Ho, H., Lazaro, R., Hua Thng, C., Yuen, J., Sing Ng, W., Cheng, C.: Optimum slicing of radical prostatectomy specimens for correlation between histopathology and medical images. Int. J. CARS **5**, 471–487 (2010)
11. Shah, V., Pohida, T., Turkbey, B., Mani, H., Merino, M., Pinto, P.A., Choyke, P., Bernardo, M.: A method for correlating in vivo prostate magnetic resonance imaging and histopathology using individualized magnetic resonance-based molds. Rev. Sci. Instrum. **80**(10), 104301 (2009)
12. Priester, A., Natarajan, S., Le, J.D., Garritano, J., Radosavcev, B., Grundfest, W., Margolis, D.J., Marks, L.S., Huang, J.: A system for evaluating magnetic resonance imaging of prostate cancer using patient-specific 3D printed molds. Am. J. Clin. Exp. Urol. **2**(2), 127–135 (2014)
13. Orczyk, C., Taneja, S.S., Rusinek, H., Rosenkrantz, A.B.: Assessment of change in prostate volume and shape following surgical resection through co-registration of in-vivo MRI and fresh specimen ex-vivo MRI. Clin. Radiol. **69**(10), 398–403 (2014)
14. Klein, S., Staring, M., Murphy, K., Viergever, M., Pluim, J.: Elastix: a toolbox for intensity based medical image registration. IEEE TMI **29**(1), 196–205 (2010)

Trajectory Smoothing for Guiding Aortic Valve Delivery with Transapical Access

Mustafa Bayraktar[1]([⊠]), Sertan Kaya[2], Erol Yeniaras[3],
and Kamran Iqbal[4]

[1] Department of Bioinformatics, UALR, Little Rock, AR 72204, USA
mxbayraktar@ualr.edu
[2] Monsanto, St. Louis, MO 65066, USA
sertankaya@monsanto.com
[3] Boeing, Houston, TX 77036, USA
eyeniaras@gmail.com
[4] Department of Systems Engineering, UALR, Little Rock, AR 72204, USA
kxiqbal@ualr.edu

Abstract. Image-guided preoperative planning is of paramount significance in obtaining reproducible results in robotic cardiac surgeries. Planning can help the surgeon utilize the derived quantitative information of the target area, and evaluate the suitability of offered medical therapy prior to surgery. In transapical aortic valve surgeries, determining the safest path for the robotic delivery module along the left ventricle (LV) is an important step to prevent potential adverse events from happening, e.g., harming inner ventricular walls and mitral valves, and malpositioning the prosthetic valve. Motivated from that fact, we processed short-axis (SAX) cardiac magnetic resonance (CMR) images which provide promising volumetric visualization with no radiation effect. More precisely, we propose a system that incorporates robust left ventricle segmentation, a combination of an isotropic denoising and a hybrid active contour model, as well as a dynamic safe path optimization for robotic delivery based on LV segments.

Keywords: Preoperative planning · MRI · Transapical Aortic Valve Replacement · Level set methods

1 Introduction

Image guidance for cardiac surgeries, especially when combined with robotic manipulation, has an ample potential to enhance efficacy of procedures. Among these procedures, Transapical Aortic Valve Implantation (TA-AVI), which is applied on beating heart, provides access to aortic root area via a small hole on the apex of the heart.

Since the last decade, real-time magnetic resonance imaging (MRI) has been used as a powerful modality for planning, guiding, and monitoring TA-AVI. MRI guidance offers certain benefits such as: (a) a wide range contrast mechanism in visualizing soft tissue, (b) no ionization radiation, (c) tracking the delivery tools, (d) real-time response to control the procedure. Based upon these advantages, potential of MRI-guided, robot-assisted TA-AVI has been demonstrated [1]. For preoperative planning of

© Springer International Publishing AG 2016
R. Shekhar et al. (Eds.): CLIP 2016, LNCS 9958, pp. 44–51, 2016.
DOI: 10.1007/978-3-319-46472-5_6

TA-AVI, a large volume of published studies focused on projecting the safest delivery that embodies the calculated angle between aorta and Left Ventricle (LV), aortic root area, the safest corridor along LV, virtual textures to reach the target area relied on different modalities [1, 2]. Among these quantitative parameters, the safest path calculation for robotic delivery module along the LV has the most critical findings in the planning stage before surgery [1–4]. Because, the dynamic safe corridor calculation is required for orienting the delivery module successfully along the determined LV corridor without damaging the heart walls and mitral valve leaflets, as well as preventing any potential adverse events during transapical access. Figure 1 illustrates a transapical access aortic valve replacement.

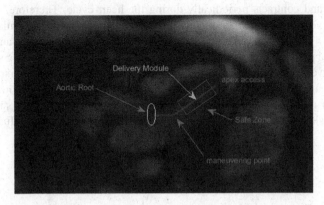

Fig. 1. A real time long axis (LAX) cardiac MR image shows transapical access to off-pump heart. All magenta variables are subject to change with time due to the dynamic structure of the environment. As can be seen by naked eye, real-time MR slices require being denoised.

So far, considerable amount of approaches has been proposed to calculate the safest corridor for TA-AVI. Yeniaras et al. [5] developed a method for updating an access corridor from the apex to the aortic annulus on-the-fly via registering pre-operative multislice dynamic MRI into single-slice real-time MRI. Zhou et al. [3] evaluated a Bayesian based algorithm to trace landmarks of heart, assessing of those useful for generating the safest corridor for device penetration, that are apex, medium, valve and centroid using long axis (LAX) and short axis images (SAX). However, both methods used cine-MRI, and did not consider the papillary muscles` artifact affects in high precision while determining the landmarks of heart. Bayraktar et al. [6] proposed to utilize Perona Malik [7] filtering method prior to active contours for segmenting LV over the heart cycle. Even though diffusion based filtering method helped them eliminate the artifacts, their approach lacks of validation for generating the safest path along LV. In this paper, we propose to bring two sequential novelties and an enhancement compared to former approaches [3, 5, 6] which are in the following.

- Utilizing an isotropic filtering supported by active contour modeling for accurate segmentation of LV borders [7, 8], which requires only one user intervention,

- Harvesting spatio-temporal LV border data, obtained by adaptive LV segmentation, and optimize the safest zone for the voyage of delivery module toward aortic root,
- Processing real-time gated Cardiac MRI slices, which brings robustness to our prototype in terms of dealing with noisy image acquisition during MR compatible robotic TA-AVI procedure.

2 Methodology

2.1 Left Ventricle Segmentation

LV expands and contracts periodically during the heart cycle. Therefore, we have to track the left ventricle borders on timely basis. We manually select a circular region of interest (ROI) around the center of the left ventricle on the first frame and initiate a computational process consisting of Perona-Malik filtering as the denoising step and the localized active contours method as the segmentation [8]. Center of the first segmented region is propagated over slices as the ROI, so that no more user intervention is required.

First step is to call Perona-Malik noise filtering method, in which smoothing is constrained when diffusion encounters strong edges. In other words, diffusivity 'g' is modeled as,

$$g(\nabla(u)) = \frac{1}{1 + \sqrt{1 + \frac{\nabla u^2}{\gamma^2}}} \tag{1}$$

This equation implies that g is inversely proportional to the image gradient ∇u of which norm serves as edge indicator, $|\nabla u| = \sqrt{u_x^2 + u_y^2}$. u represents the given image and u_x, u_y are spatial components. γ is a constant and controls the sensitivity to image gradients. Diffusion process will not affect the regions where $|\nabla u| \gg \gamma$. Note that, since g is scalar therefore this filtering must be described as isotropic, however it is still non-linear.

Second step involves in segmenting LV. We have adopted Lankton method which incorporates local image statistics into Chan-Vese energy minimization formula and let curves deform via this energy to extract object outlines despite intensity inhomogeneity in the boundary of LV and existence of papillary muscles. To perform that, a cost function along the initialized curve (which is to evolve) is constructed. This function is to approximate intensity means in the vicinity of all points on the curve. Here, vicinity is defined by a ball which is divided by the curve border into two, as the part falls in the curve called interior, and the rest part is called exterior. Energy definition is given in the following equation,

$$E = \oint_{C(S)} \int_{x \in \Omega} (I_m(p, s) - u_l(s))^2 + \int_{x \in \bar{\Omega}} (I_m(p, s) - v_l(s))^2 ds \tag{2}$$

where, Ω and $\bar{\Omega}$ represent the interior and exterior region in sequence. Curve is parametrized by 's' to specify each points on the initial curve as its integral is computed. p is a point on the curve. u_l and v_l are the arithmetic means of the pixels in the vicinity of the point on the curve. m refers to the characteristic function which is to create these local masks by evaluating 1 on the neighborhoods, and 0 elsewhere. Due to the line integral over different regions, minimization of this equation is not a straight forward process and involves in variational calculus. Hence, we refer the interested readers to [7] for more details. Figure 2 shows the contribution of Perona-Malik filtering to the curve evolution along the LV outline.

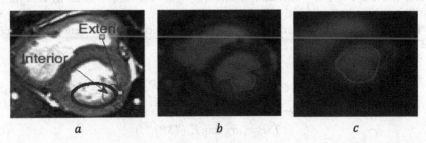

a b c

Fig. 2. (a) Represents exterior and interior Image Forces for setting the energy equation of segmentation method on SA MR, (b) represents the difficulty of handling intensity inhomogeneity during curve evolution (c) Papillary muscles are denoised by Perona Malik method before level set segmentation. Note that, in (b) and (c) midventricle slices on which papillary muscles are visible, are used for comparison. We observe that while the noise on the slices has been removed, i.e., papillary muscles, the left ventricle borders are strictly preserved. Therefore, segmentation algorithm results in more accurate delineation especially on the mid-ventricle slices.

2.2 Path Optimization

Cardiac SAX slices are parallel to each other, and collected with the same field of view. Additionally, the area from apex of the heart to the base can be densely imaged on SA view. This property of SAX view leads us to conduct the following steps that have been propagated over every single heart cycle (t = 1 to 25) and slices (s = 1 to 7) in order to determine the safest path. After user intervenes on the first slice to place the initial curve, segmented 2D contours that are specific polygons, are concatenated along z axis within a certain distance, that information can be obtained from DICOM metadata, and d + t model of LV has been created, Centroid of 2D contours is calculated by the following equations

$$C_x(t) = \frac{1}{6A} \sum_{s=1}^{7} (x_s + x_{s+1}) + (x_s y_{s+1} - x_{s+1} y_s) \qquad (3)$$

$$C_y(t) = \frac{1}{6A} \sum_{s=1}^{7} (y_s + y_{s+1}) + (x_s y_{s+1} - x_{s+1} y_s) \qquad (4)$$

In Eqs. (3) and (4); x and y are the scanned pixel coordinate values by the segmented contours (polygons) on the image plane, and A is signed area of the contours, and computed by a triangle method, that can also be used for validating the segmentation results. s represents the number of spatial layers and these two equations are run for each time frame, which is t and varies arbitrarily from 1 to 25. The reason behind calculating the centroids is that we propose that only if a sufficient distance to the heart walls is maintained, necessary condition for the safest path will be met. This can be achieved by forcing the delivery module to penetrate via the centroids of cropped segments. Nevertheless, it is desired that delivery modules are designed with less joints, so that feasible trajectory (including maneuvering points) needs to be as straight as possible and not to be abruptly cornered as shown Fig. 1. Under these constraints, in the Eq. (5) we propose to perform a spatial optimization over the dense SAX slices ($s = 7$) and time frames ($t = 25$) of a heart cycle.

$$E_\lambda(TSP) = \frac{1}{2}\sum_{s=1}^{7}(Centroids - TSP)^2 + \frac{\lambda}{2}\sum_{s=1}^{7}(TSP_{s+1} - TSP_s)^2 \tag{5}$$

$$TSP = arg\min_{TSP} E_\lambda(TSP) \tag{6}$$

First term refers how much the safest path TSP converges to the centroids, and second term is the smoothness term which makes TSP function be spatially smooth to avoid sudden zigzags on the trajectory. The λ is the weight term that controls the tendency of trajectory between the designated constrains. Since Eq. (5) is strictly convex, minimization can be performed by taking derivative of E_λ with respect to TSP. Equation (5) should be solved in two dimensions and repeated for every time frame. Figure 3 illustrates the path generation over the heart cycle.

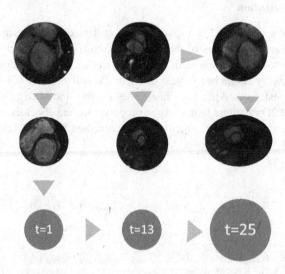

Fig. 3. The first and the third column represent end diastolic phase, and the second represents end systolic phase. First row shows base and second row shows apex of the heart in SAX view. Note that 5 mid slices were not placed due to space limitations.

3   Data Sets and Experimental Results

The data is multi-slice non-triggered and free-breathing imaging, which was performed with a true fast imaging with steady-state precession (TrueFISP), at a T_{ACQ} = 70.50 ms per slice (Pixel Spacing: 1.25 × 1.25; FOV: 299 × 399; TR: 70.50 ms; TE: 1.03 ms; Matrix: 192*72; and Slice Thickness: 8 mm). The computational core was implemented on a dedicated PC (Intel 2.5 GHz processor with 8 GB RAM). Data set consists of 165 short axis CMR slices.

3.1   LV Segmentation Validation

The performance of our segmentation method is evaluated by using two metrics, i.e., the Jaccard index, and the cross correlation between our automatic segmentation and the ground truth. The ground truth is obtained by manual delineation of the heart cavity border by an expert MRI interpreter. In order to present the enhancement of our segmentation approach, we compared our results with the results of [7], that performs only Gaussian filtering in the preprocessing phase, and Chan-Vese [8] approach that depends only on the global intensity information of the images. We selected γ as 30 when performing filtering, which controls the diffusion conduction. This value is determined empirically so that it suits for our data set (Table 1).

Table 1. Comparison of the proposed approach, and the methods in [7, 8] to manual segmentation. Correlation coefficients signifies the similarity between two crops in pixel-wise. Mean/std represents the mean and standard deviation of the comparisons between automatically segmented region and manually contoured region for each metric.

Approach	Correlation (Mean + Std)	Jaccard (Mean + Std)
Ours	0.95 ± 0.0029	0.8958 ± 0.0152
Lankton	0.93 ± 0.00187	0.8914 ± 0.0138
Chan-Vese	0.9436 ± 0.0061	0.7378 ± 0.0202

3.2   Trajectory Validation

We used Hausdorff distance to compare the trajectories, found by the method described herein, to the manually defined ground truth. Hausdorff measures distance between two subsets of a metric domain. Table 2 shows the validation results. Our method outperformed the other trajectory planning and LV tracking methods which can be categorized in active contours models (refer to Table 2). We selected λ as 0.4 and used fit function provided by MATLAB to smooth our spline-like trajectory. This command minimizes the energy by the Levenberg-Marquardt method which deploys a search direction that is a cross between the direction of steepest descent and Gauss-Newton. As mentioned in the Chap. 2.2, we used centroids of the segments to determine the safest path. We also compared our results with one of the previous method [4]. Figure 4 represents the dynamic trajectory which is subject to change.

Table 2. Hausdorff distances for each time frame and spatial slices are computed and their max/mean and minimum values are noted. Therefore, these values are the statistical variables of 7 spatial slices and 25 time frames. First, we have taken maximum, minimum and the mean values of the 25 distances for each spatial slices. Therefore, we obtained 21 statistical values for 7 slices. Then, we have calculated maximum, minimum and mean values of these values which are displayed in the table.

Method	Max	Min	Mean
Chan-Vese Based LV Tracking	1.8018	0.3182	0.992
Lankton Based LV Tracking	2.2645	0.3554	1.2273
Yeniaras et al.	2.1583	1.847	2
Ours	1.4036	0.1925	0.7692

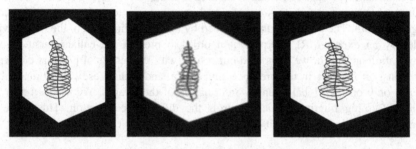

Fig. 4. Figure represents the dynamic safest path which is subject to change during systole and diastole period; it is shown in cyan color [5]. (Color figure online)

4   Discussion

We introduced a new computational preoperative planning methodology for performing real-time Transapical Aortic Valve Replacement in beating heart. The method extracts cavity borders using a refined active contour model and constructs 3d + t LV structure by projecting them onto a virtual plane along their common orthogonal axis. Cavity border delineation is performed by a specific algorithm architecture that is to facilitate processing on extremely noisy MR slices and weak edges suffer from higher intensity inhomogeneity. Volumetric depth of the 4d structure can give an idea about the maximum size of the delivery module to be used. Additionally, based on spatiotemporal analysis of the LV model, we optimized a dynamic safe path, updating it with time, and assessment of the anatomical structure of LV. The main advantage of optimizing trajectory is to make the path planning immune to even "not so accurate" segmentation results. The quantitative information provided by our approach can be transferred to world coordinates and transmitted to intraprocedure step via a structured DICOM. Nevertheless, breakdown point of our approach is that during the procedure if patient`s relative orientation to imaging equipment is different from the preoperative scan, reported trajectory might slightly tilt from where it should be. To this end, future work contains performing the experiments over various scanning techniques (within MRI) to broaden our prototype for supporting anticipated artifacts due to imaging.

References

1. Yeniaras, E., Lamaury, J., Navkar, N.V., Shah, D.J., Chin, K., Deng, Z., Tsekos, N.V.: Magnetic resonance based control of a robotic manipulator for interventions in the beating heart. In: IEEE International Conference of Robotics and Automation, pp. 6270–6275 (2011)
2. Navkar, N.V., Yeniaras, E., Shah, D.J., Tsekos, N.V., Deng, Z.: Generation of 4D access corridors from real-time multislice mri for guiding transapical aortic valvuloplasties. In: Fichtinger, G., Martel, A., Peters, T. (eds.) MICCAI 2011, Part I. LNCS, vol. 6891, pp. 251–258. Springer, Heidelberg (2011)
3. Zhou, Y., Yeniaras, E., Tsiamyrtzism, P., Tsekos, N., Pavlidis, I.: Collaborative tracking for MRI-guided robotic intervention on the beating heart. In: Jiang, T., Navab, N., Pluim, J.P.W., Viergever, M.A. (eds.) MICCAI 2010, Part III. LNCS, vol. 6363, pp. 351–358. Springer, Heidelberg (2010)
4. Yeniaras, E., Navkar, N.V., Sonmez, A.E., Shah, D.J., Deng, Z., Tsekos, N.V.: MR-based real time path planning for cardiac operations with transapical access. In: Fichtinger, G., Martel, A., Peters, T. (eds.) MICCAI 2011, Part I. LNCS, vol. 6891, pp. 25–32. Springer, Heidelberg (2011)
5. Bayraktar, M., Sahin, B., Yeniaras, E., Iqbal, K.: Applying an active contour model for pre-operative planning of transapical aortic valve replacement. In: Linguraru, M.G., Laura, C. O., Shekhar, R., Wesarg, S., Ballester, M.Á.G., Drechsler, K., Sato, Y., Erdt, M. (eds.) CLIP 2014. LNCS, vol. 8680, pp. 151–158. Springer, Heidelberg (2014)
6. Perona, P., Malik, J.: Scale-space and edge detection using anisotropic difussion. IEEE Trans. Pattern Anal. Mach. Intell. 12(7), 629–639 (1990)
7. Lankton, S., Tannebaum, A.: Localizing region-based active contours. IEEE Trans. Image Process. 17(11), 2029–2039 (2008)
8. Chan, T.F., Vese, L.A.: Active contour without edges. IEEE Trans. Image Process. 10(2), 266–277 (2011)

Geodesic Registration for Cervical Cancer Radiotherapy

Sharmili Roy[1]([✉]), John J. Totman[1], Joseph Ng[2], Jeffrey Low[2],
and Bok A. Choo[2]

[1] A*Star-NUS Clinical Imaging Research Centre, Singapore, Singapore
sharmili@nuhs.edu.sg
[2] National University Cancer Institute, Singapore, Singapore

Abstract. Uterus, bladder and rectum are the maximally exposed organs during cervical cancer radiotherapy and are at high risk of radiation exposure. Estimation of dose accumulation in these organs across multiple fractions of external beam radiotherapy (EBRT) and brachytherapy (BT) is extremely challenging due to structural mis-correspondences and complex anatomical deformations between the EBRT and BT images. This paper proposes a unified registration framework that aligns multiple EBRT and BT images of a patient to a single coordinate frame for a cumulative dose assessment. The proposed method transforms the radiotherapy anatomical images to their distance maps from the critical organs (uterus, bladder, and rectum) and registers the distance maps. A Markov random field model is used to fuse the resulting dense deformations and transform the anatomical image. Registration accuracy is evaluated on 42 clinical image pairs and it is shown that the proposed system outperforms existing methods in the literature.

Keywords: Brachytherapy · Dose accumulation · Cervical cancer · Geodesic registration

1 Introduction

Radiotherapy has proven to be very effective for cervical cancer treatment. Concurrent weekly chemotherapy, external beam radiotherapy (EBRT) and high-dose-rate brachytherapy (BT) is the standard treatment strategy for locally advanced cervical cancer. Brachytherapy, many a times in multiple fractions, is used to augment EBRT. Treatment outcome highly depends on organ doses over multiple treatment fractions [1]. Treatment evaluation should, therefore, consider the combined EBRT and BT dose in each tissue over all sessions. In current clinical practices, however, each treatment fraction is optimized independently resulting in multiple dose distributions correlated with their corresponding anatomical images. The anatomical images are collected at different points in time and exhibit large anatomical variations. Accurate registration of the underlying anatomical images is essential for dose accumulation [2]. Many factors make this registration very challenging. The brachytherapy applicator and

© Springer International Publishing AG 2016
R. Shekhar et al. (Eds.): CLIP 2016, LNCS 9958, pp. 52–59, 2016.
DOI: 10.1007/978-3-319-46472-5_7

the bladder balloon used for brachytherapy delivery introduce missing structural correspondences between EBRT and BT images and cause complicated anatomical deformations. Differences in rectum and bladder filling and tumor shrinkage with treatment are also factors that magnify registration difficulties.

A recent study on EBRT to BT dose mapping using intensity-based non-rigid registration available on a commercial software report that registration failed in 40 % patients due to 'unreasonable' anatomical deformations [2]. Four papers have presented algorithms for registration between EBRT and BT images [1,3,4] or between two BT images [5] using customized registration routines. The first attempted approach was to use a viscous fluid model and transform the EBRT image to the BT image without using any bio-mechanical models [1]. Multiple runs of the algorithm were often required to achieve satisfactory results. Recently, Berendsen et al. [3] proposed a geometric penalty-based registration that folds the applicator region and brings its volume to zero. This algorithm assumes that an applicator model is always available before each registration. Applicators are typically chosen and installed according to a patient's uterus/cervix size prior to every fraction. Creating an applicator model before each session is clinically impractical. Osorio et al. [4] segment various tube-like and sheet-like features surrounding the critical organs and independently register each pair of features and each pair of critical organs. Composition of the individual registrations gives a final deformation vector. No regularization constraints the underlying registrations to be coherent. Another paper by Zhen et al. [5] registers BT image pairs by segmenting the applicator region in both fixed and moving images and matching surface points on the cavity left by the segmented applicators. This method is very accurate in matching the applicator volume, however, organ-based registration accuracies are not reported.

These existing studies focus either only on (EBRT,BT) image pairs or only on (BT,BT) image pairs. No published algorithm, to the best of our knowledge, can register any combination of EBRT and BT images within the same framework. This paper proposes such a unified framework that registers any combination of radiotherapy images with respect to the main organs at risk (uterus, bladder, rectum). This enables assessment of the total dose received over all EBRT and BT sessions while a patient is still undergoing treatment. The ultimate goal of this research is to empower personalized dose painting so that radiotherapy can be fine-tuned based on an individual's response to therapy.

2   Methods

This paper presents a registration approach that is designed on a data set where the EBRT and the BT images are acquired at different clinical sites and in scanners that have different field strengths and scanning protocols. No assumptions are made regarding the deformation of the individual organs. As a first step in the registration pipeline, the fixed and the moving gray-level images are registered using a mutual information based affine transformation. The fixed image for (EBRT,BT) pair registration is the BT image and the moving image is the

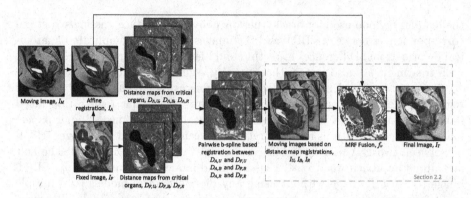

Fig. 1. Overview of the registration pipeline. Geodesic distance maps from the critical organs are non-linearly registered. An MRF model composes these registrations and the background registration into a final transform

EBRT image. To overcome different acquisition protocols and structural dissimilarities, the anatomical images are transformed into their distance maps based on delineations of the critical organs which are assumed to be available as in similar works in the literature [1,4]. Three distance maps, one each from the uterus, the bladder and the rectum are generated for both the images. Each corresponding distance map pairs are non-linearly registered using a B-spline-based registration which is formulated with a similarity energy function comprising of mutual information [6] and a rigidity penalty [7]. Ten iterations of this registration are applied in a multi-resolution fashion where the control point spacing gradually reduces to eight voxels. Elastix toolbox is used for implementation of this registration scheme [8]. A Markov random field (MRF) model, detailed in Sect. 2.2, is used to combine the distance-map and the background registrations (Fig. 1).

2.1   Distance Map Computation

A recent study by Roy et al. show that geodesic distance is better than traditional physical distances for registration in cervical cancer [9]. Geodesic distances take into account image gradients and characterize distances using the shortest path along the image gradients [11]. Given a 3D image I, an anatomical region Ω, and a binary mask M (with $M(\boldsymbol{x}) \in \{0,1\}\ \forall \boldsymbol{x}$ such that $\boldsymbol{x} \in \Omega \Longleftrightarrow M(\boldsymbol{x}) = 0$, the unsigned geodesic distance of each voxel $\boldsymbol{x}$ from Ω is defined as:

$$D(\boldsymbol{x}; M, \nabla I) = \min_{\{\boldsymbol{x}' \mid M(\boldsymbol{x}') = 0\}} d(\boldsymbol{x}, \boldsymbol{x}'), \tag{1}$$

$$d(\boldsymbol{a}, \boldsymbol{b}) = \min_{\boldsymbol{\Gamma} \in \mathcal{P}_{\boldsymbol{a},\boldsymbol{b}}} \int_0^{l(\boldsymbol{\Gamma})} \sqrt{1 + \gamma^2 (\nabla I(s) \cdot \boldsymbol{\Gamma}'(s))^2}\ ds, \tag{2}$$

with $\mathcal{P}_{\boldsymbol{a},\boldsymbol{b}}$ being the set of all possible differentiable paths between points $\boldsymbol{a}$ and $\boldsymbol{b}$. $\boldsymbol{\Gamma}(s): \Re \to \Re^3$ represents such a path parametrized by its arclength $s \in [0, l(\boldsymbol{\Gamma}))]$. The spatial derivative $\boldsymbol{\Gamma}'(s) = \partial \boldsymbol{\Gamma}(s)/\partial s$ is tangent to the path direction. γ controls the contribution of the image gradient with respect to the physical distances and for $\gamma = 0, D$ reduces to Euclidean distance.

2.2   Markov Random Field Fusion

Fusing multiple registrations of an image pair using MRF is known to yield high accuracy [10]. We formulate registration fusion as a labeling problem where the goal is to find the best registration for each voxel. The four registrations to choose from are the background affine registration and the three non-linear distance map registrations. Let $I_F(\boldsymbol{x}) : \Omega_F$ and $I_M(\boldsymbol{x}) : \Omega_M$ be the fixed and the moving anatomical images with domains $\Omega_F, \Omega_M \subset \mathbb{R}^3$ respectively. The affine registered image, $I_A = I_M(T_A(\boldsymbol{x})) : \Omega_F$, is obtained by interpolating I_M at the affine transformed voxel coordinates of I_F. Let $D_{F,U}$ and $D_{A,U}$ be the uterus-based distance maps of I_F and I_A respectively. The distance maps $D_{F,U}$ and $D_{A,U}$ are registered using a B-spline transformation model $T_\mu(\boldsymbol{x})$ with coefficients μ. The resulting dense deformation is used to transform I_A and compute $I_U = T_\mu(I_A)$. Similarly, $D_{F,B}$, $D_{A,B}$ and $D_{F,R}$, $D_{A,R}$ are defined as the bladder-based and rectum-based distance maps of I_F and I_A respectively. The images I_B and I_R are computed by registering the bladder-based and the rectum-based distance maps and transforming I_A respectively (refer Fig. 1).

Let I_T be the final transformed image. The labeling problem assigns each voxel $v \in V$, a registration that minimizes the disagreement between $I_F(v)$ and $I_T(v)$. The label set consists of the four registrations that are assigned labels U for uterus-based, B for bladder-based, R for rectum-based and A for the background affine registration. The goal is to find a labeling function f that assigns a $f_v \in \{U, B, R, A\}, \forall v \in V$ such that the following objective function $E(f)$ is minimized:

$$E(f) = \sum_{v \in V} \mathcal{V}_v(f_v) + \sum_{u \in N_v} \mathcal{V}_{uv}(f_u, f_v), \tag{3}$$

where $\mathcal{V}_u$ measures the difference between $I_{f_v}(v)$ and $I_F(v)$ and $\mathcal{V}_{uv}$ penalizes $f_u \neq f_v$ for all neighbors N_v of v. Each voxel v is connected to 26 neighbors in the 3D space. We use the Potts model for the pairwise potential defined as $\mathcal{V}(x, y) = K \cdot T(x \neq y)$, where $T(\cdot)$ is 1 if its argument is true, and 0 otherwise. The data term, $\mathcal{V}_v$, is defined as:

$$\mathcal{V}_v(f_v) = \frac{1}{|N_v| + 1} \sum_{u \in (N_v \cup v)} (I_F(u) - I_{f_v}(u))^2 + \alpha D_{A, f_v}(v) \cdot T(f_v \neq A), \tag{4}$$

where α weighs the voxel's geodesic distance from the corresponding critical organ. Geodesic distances are less accurate as the voxel moves further away from the organ surface. The second term in Eq. 4 increases the energy if the voxel is too far away from the organ on which the distance map and the registration is based. Since the background affine transformation is not dependent on any organ or distance transformation, $D_{A,A}$ is not defined and hence excluded from the second term. The solution of Eq. 3 gives a voxel-wise registration map that is used to compose the final image as $I_T(v) = I_{f_v}(v), \forall v \in V$.

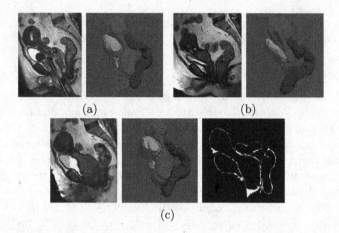

Fig. 2. (EBRT,BT) registration. (a) Fixed BT image (I_F) and the critical organ delineations on I_F. Blue, red and gray colors are for uterus, rectum and bladder respectively. (b) Moving EBRT image (I_M) and the organ delineations. (c) The registered image (I_T), propagated organ delineations and their absolute difference with ground truth on I_F. Higher intensities show higher differences (Color figure online)

Table 1. This table compares the mean registration accuracy of the proposed method with Osorio et al. [4] and Berendsen et al. [3] for (EBRT,BT) registration. Mean Hausdorff distances (HD) in mm and Dice coefficients are compared

Anatomy	Osorio et al. (Mean shortest dist.)	Berendsen et al. (Dice coeff.)	Ours (HD/Dice coeff.)	Masked Reg. (HD/Dice coeff.)
Uterus	1.60	0.77	**0.67/0.88**	6.67/0.40
Bladder	1.25	0.75	**0.30/0.91**	3.58/0.50
Rectum	1.15	0.78	**1.00/0.82**	4.21/0.44

3   Results

42 image pairs from clinical stage 2B−4A cervical cancer patients are used to assess the registration accuracy. The BT and EBRT images are acquired on 1.5T Magnetic Resonance (MR) and 3T simultaneous positron emission technology/magnetic resonance (PET/MR) machines respectively. In some cases EBRT and BT images are acquired three months apart. Figure 2 illustrates a (EBRT,BT) image pair registration and it is observed that the proposed method successfully handles large deformations in the critical organs. Table 1 compares the mean registration accuracy of (EBRT,BT) pairs with those reported in related works and shows that the presented framework outperforms existing methods. The Dice coefficients and the Hausdorff distances are computed between the organ delineations on the fixed image and the propagated delineations on the registered image. Since the registration is driven by the critical organ labels, it seems that a direct registration between images multiplied by their corresponding critical masks might

Table 2. This table lists the registration accuracy in terms of mean Dice coefficient for (BT,BT) and (EBRT,EBRT) image pairs

Image pair	Uterus	Bladder	Rectum
(BT,BT)	0.93	0.91	0.83
(EBRT,EBRT)	0.84	0.87	0.63

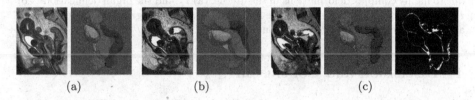

| (a) | (b) | (c) |

Fig. 3. (BT,BT) registration. (a) Fixed BT image and the organ delineations. (b) Moving BT image and the organ delineations. (c) The registered image, propagated organ delineations and their absolute difference with ground truth

also work. The last column reports accuracy when masked images are directly registered using a B-spline-based registration.

Other image pairs such as (BT,BT) and (EBRT,EBRT) can also be registered within the proposed framework. Figure 3 illustrates a (BT,BT) image registration and Table 2 shows mean accuracy for (BT,BT) and (EBRT,EBRT) pairs. A comparison of performance with existing methods could not be done because Berendsen et al. [3] and Osorio et al. [4] target only (EBRT,BT) pairs and Zhen et al. [5] do not report uterus level registration accuracy for (BT,BT) pairs. To the best of our knowledge, this is the first registration pipeline that can handle all combinations of EBRT and BT images within the same framework. For cases when the patient has an anteverted (forward tilted) uterus, the complexity of deformation is much higher and the registration accuracy is lower (Fig. 4). An anteverted uterus shows more complex deformations as the tumor shrinks with treatment making (EBRT,EBRT) registration also very challenging.

Table 3 shows that fusion achieves higher accuracy for all critical organs than registrations that are based on only one critical organ. For all experiments, the parameter α in Eq. 4 is set to one. Experimentally we observe that the registration accuracy is fairly insensitive to α.

Table 3. This table compares registration accuracy of MRF fusion with registrations based on individual critical organs for (EBRT,BT) image pairs in terms of Dice coefficients

Anatomy	Uterus-based reg.	Bladder-based reg.	Rectum-based reg	MRF fusion
Uterus	0.88	0.49	0.45	0.88
Bladder	0.63	0.90	0.54	0.91
Rectum	0.60	0.54	0.85	0.82

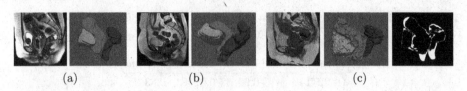

(a)   (b)   (c)

Fig. 4. (EBRT,BT) registration for an anteverted uterus. Registration accuracy is lower due to highly complex deformations in the uterus. (a) I_F and the organ delineations. (b) I_M and the organ delineations. (c) The registered image, propagated organ delineations and their absolute difference with ground truth

4   Discussion and Conclusion

This paper addresses the problem of registering radiotherapy MR images of the pelvis for quantifying dose accumulation in critical organs across BT and EBRT sessions. Traditional deformable registration methods fail to handle the complex deformations present in these images. The paper advocates the use of geodesic distance maps that can be more robustly registered than the original anatomical images. Converting anatomical images to distance maps effectively simplifies the registration challenges and allows to register a pair of EBRT images or a pair of BT images or a combination of EBRT and BT images within the same registration scheme. The idea is to be able to transfer organ locations/delineations from one treatment day to the other for a personalized and adaptive planning of radiotherapy. We believe that the idea of registering distance maps from critical organs can also be used for registration and dose accumulation during radiotherapy of other cancers in the pelvis such as prostate and rectum. Evaluation of the method for rectal cancer dose accumulation is under investigation.

The proposed method assumes apriori critical organ delineations. Typically in MRI-guided radiation therapy planning for cervical cancer, the tumor, cervix, vagina, uterus, bladder and rectum are circumscribed in MR images by a radiation therapist [12]. In theory, this existing data can be used for registration if accessible. Further, in future we plan to study the sensitivity of registration with respect to segmentation accuracy and investigate the use of semi-automated/automated segmentation.

A limitation of this work is that MRF fusion cannot guarantee smoothness at the label 'seams', potentially leading to folding in the transformation. Competing methods also suffer from this problem. We are currently investigating Gaussian smoothing as suggested in [10] for folding removal as a post-processing step. In addition, we are working on evaluating the method using a landmark based approach where anatomically relevant landmarks will be placed on and in-between the critical organs. By doing this, we can quantify the accuracy of the dense deformation field and also compute the dose volume histograms which is a more powerful tool for dose accumulation.

Acknowledgment. The work is partially funded by NMRC NUHS Centre Grant Medical Image Analysis Core (NMRC/CG/013/2013).

References

1. Christensen, G.E., Carlson, B., Chao, K.S.C., Yin, P., Grigsby, P.W., Nguyen, K., Dempsey, J.F., Lerma, F.A., Bae, K.T., Vannier, M.W., et al.: Image-based dose planning of intracavitary brachytherapy: registration of serial-imaging studies using deformable anatomic templates. Int. J. Rad. Oncol. Biol. Phys. **51**(1), 227–243 (2001)
2. Kim, H., Huq, M.S., Houser, C., Beriwal, S., Michalski, D.: Mapping of dose distribution from IMRT onto MRI-guided high dose rate brachytherapy using deformable image registration for cervical cancer treatments: preliminary study with commercially available software. J. Contemp. Brachyther. **6**(2), 178–184 (2014)
3. Berendsen, F.F., Kotte, A.N.T.J., de Leeuw, A.A.C., Jürgenliemk-Schulz, I.M., Viergever, M.A., Pluim, J.P.W.: Registration of structurally dissimilar images in MRI-based brachytherapy. Phys. Med. Biol. **59**(15), 4033 (2014)
4. Osorio, E.M.V., Kolkman-Deurloo, I.-K.K., Schuring-Pereira, M., Zolnay, A., Heijmen, B.J.M., Hoogeman, M.S.: Improving anatomical mapping of complexly deformed anatomy for external beam radiotherapy and brachytherapy dose accumulation in cervical cancer. Med. Phys. **42**(1), 206–220 (2015)
5. Zhen, X., Chen, H., Yan, H., Zhou, L., Mell, L.K., Yashar, C.M., Jiang, S., Jia, X., Gu, X., Cervino, L.: A segmentation and point-matching enhanced efficient deformable image registration method for dose accumulation between HDR CT images. Phys. Med. Biol. **60**(7), 2981 (2015)
6. Mattes, D., Haynor, D.R., Vesselle, H., Lewellyn, T.K., Eubank, W.: Nonrigid multimodality image registration. Med. Imag. **22**, 1609–1620 (2001)
7. Staring, M., Klein, S., Pluim, J.P.W.: A rigidity penalty term for nonrigid registration. Med. Phys. **34**(11), 4098–4108 (2007)
8. Klein, S., Staring, M., Murphy, K., Viergever, M., Pluim, J.P.W.: others: Elastix: a toolbox for intensity-based medical image registration. IEEE Trans. Med. Imaging **29**(1), 196–205 (2010)
9. Roy, S., Totman, J.J., Choo, B.A.: Unified registration framework for cumulative dose assessment in cervical cancer across external beam radiotherapy and brachytherapy. Proc. SPIE Med. Imaging 2016 Image Process. **9784**, 978441-1–978441-6 (2016)
10. Gass, T., Szekely, G., Goksel, O.: Registration fusion using markov random fields. In: Ourselin, S., Modat, M. (eds.) WBIR 2014. LNCS, vol. 8545, pp. 213–222. Springer, Heidelberg (2014)
11. Wang, Z., Bhatia, K.K., Glocker, B., Marvao, A., Dawes, T., Misawa, K., Mori, K., Rueckert, D.: Geodesic patch-based segmentation. In: Golland, P., Hata, N., Barillot, C., Hornegger, J., Howe, R. (eds.) MICCAI 2014, Part I. LNCS, vol. 8673, pp. 666–673. Springer, Heidelberg (2014)
12. Ghose, S., Holloway, L., Lim, K., Chan, P., Veera, J., Vinod, S.K., Liney, G., Greer, P.B., Dowling, J.: A review of segmentation and deformable registration methods applied to adaptive cervical cancer radiation therapy treatment planning. Artif. Intell. Med. **64**(2), 75–87 (2015)

Personalized Optimal Planning for the Surgical Correction of Metopic Craniosynostosis

Antonio R. Porras[1(✉)], Dženan Zukic[2], Andinet Equobahrie[2],
Gary F. Rogers[3], and Marius George Linguraru[1,4]

[1] Sheikh Zayed Institute for Pediatric Surgical Innovation,
Children's National Health System, Washington, DC, USA
aporraspe@childrensnational.org
[2] Kitware Inc., Carrboro, NC, USA
[3] Division of Plastic and Reconstructive Surgery,
Children's National Health System, Washington, DC, USA
[4] School of Medicine and Health Sciences, George Washington,
Washington, DC, USA

Abstract. We introduce a quantitative and automated method for personalized cranial shape remodeling via fronto-orbital advancement surgery. This paper builds on an objective method for automatic quantification of malformations caused by metopic craniosynostosis in children and presents a framework for personalized interventional planning. First, skull malformations are objectively quantified using a statistical atlas of normal cranial shapes. Then, we propose a method based on poly-rigid image registration that takes into account both the clinical protocol for fronto-orbital advancement and the physical constraints in the skull to plan the creation of the optimal post-surgical shape. Our automated surgical planning technique aims to minimize cranial malformations. The method was used to calculate the optimal shape for 11 infants with age 3.8 ± 3.0 month old presenting metopic craniosynostosis and cranial malformations. The post-surgical cranial shape provided for each patient presented a significant average malformation reduction of 49 % in the frontal cranial bones, and achieved shapes whose malformations were within healthy ranges. To our knowledge, this is the first work that presents an automatic framework for an objective and personalized surgical planning for craniosynostosis treatment.

Keywords: Craniosynostosis · Interventional planning · Image registration · Fronto-orbital advancement

1 Introduction

Craniosynostosis is a condition affecting 1 of every 2100–2500 [1] live births in which one or more cranial sutures fuse prematurely. In many cases, this results in an abnormal growth pattern of the cranial bones and malformations. If untreated, craniosynostosis can cause increased intra-cranial pressure, impaired brain growth, visual problems and cognitive delay [2].

Depending on which cranial suture is prematurely fused, craniosynostosis can be classified as sagittal, coronal, lambdoid or metopic. Furthermore, sometimes

© Springer International Publishing AG 2016
R. Shekhar et al. (Eds.): CLIP 2016, LNCS 9958, pp. 60–67, 2016.
DOI: 10.1007/978-3-319-46472-5_8

craniosynostosis can involve more than one suture. The case of metopic craniosynostosis is particularly challenging to diagnose, since the metopic suture fuses early in healthy subjects and, therefore, suture fusion alone is not an indicator of pathology. Studying the degree of malformation is then essential to assess metopic craniosynostosis and to decide if surgical intervention is necessary.

Fronto-orbital advancement [3] is a widely used interventional approach to correct for metopic craniosynostosis. During this intervention, the surgeon removes the frontal cranial bones and advances them forward to create a "normal" head shape with sufficient space to allow for healthy brain growth, as shown in Fig. 1. However, how to create a normal cranial shape remains a subjective surgical art.

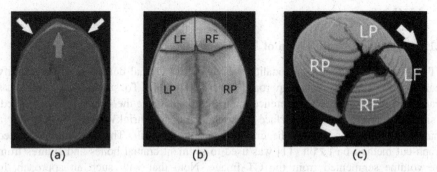

Fig. 1. Metopic craniosynostosis and fronto-orbital advancement. (a) Axial plane view of the CT image on one patient with metopic craniosynostosis. White arrows show major areas with malformations. The orange arrow shows ridging on the fused metopic suture. (b) Cranial volume of the patient in (a) extracted from CT, together with its closest normal shape (green) estimated as in [4]. The coronal sutures are delineated in blue and the fused metopic suture is shown in red. (c) Representation of the personalized optimal shape to target during a fronto-orbital advancement intervention, where the left (LF) and right frontal (RF) bones are advanced forward with respect to the left (LP) and right parietal (RP) bones. (Color figure online)

There is a lack of objective methods to quantify cranial malformations in clinical practice, which makes diagnosis, the decision to go for a surgery, and the intervention planning very dependent on the surgeon's expertise. Mendoza et al. [4] proposed a method to quantify malformations objectively from CT images using a statistical atlas. In our work, we focus on the specific case of metopic craniosynostosis, and we base on the method to quantify malformations from [4] to address the problem of creating the optimal post-surgical shape via fronto-orbital advancement surgery.

Some previous works have addressed the need of interventional planning for fronto-orbital advancement. However, most reported techniques are based on free-hand approaches for advancing the lateral supraorbital region [5, 6]. Other works [7, 8] proposed the use of a set of predefined templates and computer aided design software packages to plan fronto-orbital advancement interventions. However, none of these approaches solved the problem of objectively finding a personalized and optimal shape to target during the intervention, since they were based on subjective assessment of malformations. In addition, manual human interaction was necessary in all these works and the results were still very dependent on the specialist.

Our automated method employs image registration through a novel and invertible poly-rigid transformation inspired by [9]. Importantly, our technique incorporates the concept of purely rigid regions within the clinical protocol for fronto-orbital advancement surgery to create the optimal personalized cranial shape to target during cranial shape remodeling. In addition, it does not only provide the surgeon with a shape to target during the intervention, but it also calculates how much each bone has to be displaced during the intervention in mm. To our knowledge, this is the first time a fully automatic and objective method is proposed for fronto-orbital advancement planning.

2 Methods

2.1 Objective Quantification of Malformations

CT is the standard imaging modality used to assess cranial deformities. To quantify malformations, we used the approach described in [4]. To summarize, a patient's cranium was registered to a reference image template. Once the volumes were aligned, a single-layered, genus-zero surface was obtained using ShrinkWrap [10], obtaining a triangular mesh representing the cranial shape as a result. Then a template-guided graph-cut method based on [11] was used to segment cranial bones and sutures from the volume segmented from the CT image. Note that with such an approach, in presence of a fused suture, the segmentation algorithm is only driven by the template and the suture is delineated as in the template. Finally, cranial malformations were quantified in relation to the closest normal shape extracted from a statistical atlas built from healthy subjects using Signed Distance Function (SDF) representations of the surfaces, thus avoiding the problems related to landmark correspondences.

2.2 Optimal Personalized Intervention Planning

In this section, we introduce a method to plan the correction of metopic craniosynostosis via fronto-orbital advancement. Finding the optimal shape to target during the intervention can be viewed as an optimization problem, where a function quantifying the degree of malformations in the patient's skull has to be minimized. We propose a solution based on image registration, where the goal is to deform the volumetric image of the subject's skull to minimize its malformations. In particular, we register the volumetric image of the subject's skull to the image of the closest normal skull in the statistical shape atlas. Our framework incorporates physical constraints, namely bone rigidity, and also constraints imposed by the clinical protocol of fronto-orbital advancement, namely that only the position of the frontal bones can be modified during surgery.

A simple solution could be to estimate a rigid transformation for each of the bones separately. Instead, we employ a global registration approach to include interactions between bones and avoid bone overlaps. In [12], a method to incorporate rigid regions to an image registration problem was proposed, while allowing other types of deformation in the rest of the image. A set of rigid transformations (one per rigid object) and a global deformable transformation were linearly combined, using distance functions applied to each object to estimate the weight of its transformation at any location in the image. Such scheme ensured the weight associated to the non-linear transformation to equal zero in the rigid regions. However, the method did not guarantee invertibility of the estimated transformation. In addition, the accuracy was limited by the refinement of the underlying grid of control points and the smoothness of the radial basis functions.

In [9], a method to estimate a global transformation by combining the speed vectors from a set of rigid transformations centered on fixed anchor points was proposed. Unlike most free-form deformation approaches, this type of poly-rigid transformations solved problems related to large movements of objects. In addition, the resulting transformation was invertible. However, although the transformation was calculated from a set of local rigid transformations, no single region in the image was constrained to present a purely rigid transformation, as required in our application.

In our work, we extend the method presented in [9] by incorporating the concept of rigid regions introduced in [12], instead of using anchor points to define rigid transformations. Unlike in [12], we avoid the constraints related to using radial basis functions to define the transformation and we propose to use smooth, continuous and differentiable weighting functions to control the transition between rigid and non-rigid regions, thus ensuring the invertibility of the transformation.

Transformation model. The speed vector at a point with coordinates x is calculated by averaging the speed vectors from each rigid transformation of an object [9]:

$$v(x,s) = \frac{\sum_{\forall i} w_i(x) v_i(x,s)}{\sum_{\forall i} w_i(x)}, \tag{1}$$

where $v_i(x,s)$ is the speed vector associated to the rigid transformation i at coordinates x and time $s \in [0,1]$, and $w_i(x)$ is the weight of that rigid transformation at location x. The speed vector associated to each rigid transformation is calculated as:

$$v_i(x,s) = t_i + A_i(x - st_i), \tag{2}$$

where t_i is the translation vector of the rigid transformation i, and A_i is a skew matrix. Equation (2) is obtained by differentiating the trajectory equation $T(x,s) = st_i + exp(sA_i)T(x,0)$. The matrix A_i is defined as the logarithm of the rotation matrix and is related to the rotation vector by the following equation [9]:

$$A_i = \begin{pmatrix} 0 & -r_z & r_y \\ r_z & 0 & -r_x \\ -r_y & r_x & 0 \end{pmatrix}, \tag{3}$$

where $r = (r_x, r_y, r_z)$ is the rotation vector. In [9], the weights $w_i(x)$ were calculated using Gaussian functions centered at each anchor point defined on the image. This approach does not allow constraining different areas of the image to be purely rigid. In addition, the weighting functions proposed in [12] would not ensure the invertibility of the transformation, since they are not differentiable at the boundary of the rigid objects.

In our implementation, the rotation of each transformation is defined to be centered on the center of mass of the rigid object associated to it. We also calculate SDFs for each of the rigid objects in the image (i.e. the cranial bones), which take negative values inside the object and positive values outside. The weight function associated with the transformation of each rigid object can then be defined using a continuous, smooth and differentiable approximation to a Heaviside step function applied to the SDF of that object:

$$w_i(x) = \frac{1}{1 + \exp(c \; SDF_i(x))},$$ (4)

where $SDF_i(x)$ is the SDF calculated for object i at coordinates x, and c is a factor defining the slope of the function at the transition point (i.e. the object boundary).

Next, we integrate the velocity at each point over time to estimate the trajectory according to the transformation model. A second-order discretization scheme was proposed in [9] by defining the following operator:

$$T^{1/N}(x, s) = x + \frac{\sum_{\forall i} w_i(x) \left(\frac{1}{N} t_i + (\exp(A_i/N) - I)(x - st_i)\right)}{\sum_{\forall i} w_i(x)},$$ (5)

where I represents the identity matrix, and N is the number of discretization subintervals. Using Eq. 5, the trajectory of a point at coordinates x can be obtained recursively from the composition of that operator at different time instants: $T(x) = T^{1/N}(., (k - 1)/N) \circ \ldots \circ T^{1/N}(x, 0)$. In our implementation, we divide the temporal interval empirically into two subintervals. Although this number of discretization intervals was enough for our goal, in applications where larger displacements can be expected, discontinuities may appear and a higher discretization level may be chosen.

Dissimilarity measure. Our application aims to minimize deformities in the subject's skull. In [4], the degree of malformation was quantified as the distance between the subject's cranial shape and the reference shape (i.e. closest normal subject). In the image domain, this translates to minimizing the pixel intensity difference between the volumetric image of the patient's cranium and the closest normal subject:

$$D(F, M) = \sum_{\forall x} (M(T(x)) - F(x))^2,$$ (6)

where M is the patient's image, and F is the closest normal subject's image.

Optimization. We used a regular gradient descent optimizer for the objective function. Given the transformation model described above, a set of parameters defining as many rigid transformations as objects (i.e. cranial bones) can be optimized. However, for the

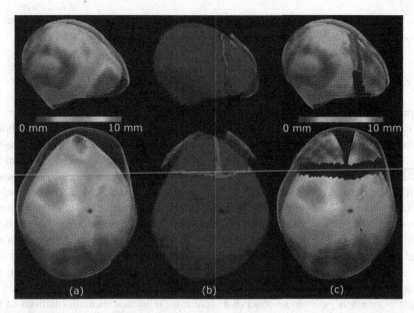

Fig. 2. Surgical planning. (a) Lateral (top) and axial (bottom) views of the malformations (color coded) estimated on one patient's skull shape, together with its closest normal shape (white wireframe). (b) Suggested cut lines (red) based on coronal and metopic sutures segmentation, together with the optimal position for the frontal bones computed with the proposed method, shown as a wireframe. (c) Malformations estimated on the optimal post-surgical shape, together with its closest normal shape (white wireframe). (Color figure online)

surgical treatment of metopic craniosynostosis via fronto-orbital advancement, only the cranial frontal bones require advancement, while the rest of the bones are kept in the same position during the intervention. For that reason, the optimization is constrained so the translation and rotation parameters of the non-frontal bones are not modified.

Evaluation. For each patient with metopic craniosynostosis, malformations were quantified using the method summarized in Sect. 2.1. After segmenting the cranial bones and sutures as in [4], we used our method to register the binary volumetric images of the patient's skull to its closest normal from the statistical atlas. The estimated transformation calculated was then applied to the subject's cranial shape to obtain the optimal shape to target during the intervention. As an example, Fig. 2 shows the interventional plan calculated for one example patient with severe metopic craniosynostosis.

2.3 Data

To create the statistical atlas of normal cranial shapes, we used axial CT images of 100 healthy infants (age 5.80 ± 3.31 months). In-plane pixel size ranged 0.26–0.49 mm, with axial spacing smaller or equal to 5 mm, in line with common clinical practice for craniosynostosis [13]. For the experiments, we used retrospective CT images from 11 subjects (age 3.8 ± 3.0 months) diagnosed with metopic craniosynostosis.

3 Results

Average malformations calculated for the 11 cases analyzed were 3.12 ± 1.38 mm for the right frontal (RF) bone and 3.34 ± 1.52 mm for the left frontal (LF) bone. A Student's t-test was used to check if these results were statistically different to the results reported in [4] for patients with metopic craniosynostosis (3.20 ± 2.07 mm for the RF bone and 2.57 ± 1.71 mm for the LF bone). Differences were not statistically significant, obtaining $p = 0.90$ and $p = 0.23$ for the RF and LF bones, respectively.

After creating the optimal post-surgical shape, malformations were significantly reduced to 1.62 ± 0.99 mm for the RF bone and 1.67 ± 0.99 mm for the LF bone ($p < 0.01$), representing an average reduction of 49 %. These values were within the range reported in [4] for healthy subjects (1.11 ± 0.63 mm for the RF bone and 1.13 ± 0.50 mm for the LF bone), with $p = 0.15$ and $p = 0.11$ for the RF and LF bones, respectively. As an example, Fig. 2 shows the interventional plan for one severe patient, where it is possible to observe a significant reduction of malformations in the frontal bones of the optimal post-surgical shape (c) with respect to the pre-operative shape (a). Note that, after the surgery, cranial bones will resume their normal growth and this will also play an important role in developing a normal skull shape.

4 Conclusions

Our technique for fronto-orbital advancement surgical planning, based on a method for an objective quantification of malformations, constitutes the first fully automatic and objective framework for metopic craniosynostosis assessment and interventional planning. We introduced a method based on image registration that takes into account bone rigidity and clinical protocol constraints, and computes a smooth and invertible transformation to reconstruct the optimal cranial shape during the intervention. We demonstrated that the post-surgical shape reconstructed with our method and the surgical plan to achieve it can significantly reduce malformations in the frontal bones by 49 %. In addition, malformations in the optimal shapes obtained were within healthy ranges. Importantly, we do not only provide the optimal shape to target during the intervention, but we also provide information about how much each bone has to be displaced and in which direction to achieve that optimal shape.

Future work includes the integration of our method in the clinical workflow for its validation. It will also be adapted to allow for bone exchange and bending, considering the mechanical properties of the bones. Finally, the versatility of this framework will allow extending it for treatment planning of other types of craniosynostosis.

Acknowledgements. This work was partly funded by the National Institutes of Health, Eunice Kennedy Shriver National Institute of Child Health and Human Development under grant NIH 1R41HD081712.

References

1. Lajeunie, E., Le Merrer, M., Bonaïti-Pellie, C., Marchac, D., Renier, D.: Genetic study of nonsyndromic coronal craniosynostosis. Am. J. Med. Genet. **55**, 500–504 (1995)
2. Wood, B.C., Mendoza, C.S., Oh, A.K., Myers, E., Safdar, N., Linguraru, M.G., Rogers, G. F.: What's in a Name? Accurately diagnosing metopic craniosynostosis using a computational approach. Plast. Reconstr. Surg. **137**, 205–213 (2016)
3. Aryan, H.E., Jandial, R., Ozgur, B.M., Hughes, S.A., Meltzer, H.S., Park, M.S., Levy, M.L.: Surgical correction of metopic synostosis. Child's Nerv. Syst. **21**, 392–398 (2005)
4. Mendoza, C.S., Safdar, N., Okada, K., Myers, E., Rogers, G.F., Linguraru, M.G.: Personalized assessment of craniosynostosis via statistical shape modeling. Med. Image Anal. **18**, 635–646 (2014)
5. Havlik, R.J., Azurin, D.J., Bartlett, S.P., Whitaker, L.A.: Analysis and treatment of severe trigonocephaly. Plast. Reconstr. Surg. **103**, 381–390 (1999)
6. Selber, J., Reid, R.R., Gershman, B., Sonnad, S.S., Sutton, L.N., Whitaker, L.A., Bartlett, S. P.: Evolution of operative techniques for the treatment of single-suture metopic synostosis. Ann. Plast. Surg. **59**, 6–13 (2007)
7. Burge, J., Saber, N.R., Looi, T., French, B., Usmani, Z., Anooshiravani, N., Kim, P., Forrest, C., Phillips, J.: Application of CAD/CAM prefabricated age-matched templates in cranio-orbital remodeling in craniosynostosis. J. Craniofac. Surg. **22**, 1810–1813 (2011)
8. Diluna, M.L., Steinbacher, D.M.: Simulated fronto-orbital advancement achieves reproducible results in metopic synostosis. J. Craniofac. Surg. **23**, 231–234 (2012)
9. Arsigny, V., Pennec, X., Ayache, N.: Polyrigid and polyaffine transformations: a novel geometrical tool to deal with non-rigid deformations - application to the registration of histological slices. Med. Image Anal. **9**, 507–523 (2005)
10. Pope, P.: Shrinkwrap: 3D model abstraction for remote sensing. In: 2009 ASPRS Annual Meeting, pp. 9–13 (2009)
11. Liu, L., Raber, D., Nopachai, D., Commean, P., Sinacore, D., Prior, F., Pless, R., Ju, T.: Interactive separation of segmented bones in CT volumes using graph cut. In: Metaxas, D., Axel, L., Fichtinger, G., Székely, G. (eds.) MICCAI 2008, Part I. LNCS, vol. 5241, pp. 296–304. Springer, Heidelberg (2008)
12. Little, J.A., Hill, D.L.G., Hawkes, D.J.: Deformations incorporating rigid structures [medical imaging]. In: Workshop on Mathematical Methods in Biomedical Image Analysis, pp. 223–232. IEEE (1996)
13. Vannier, M.W., Pilgram, T.K., Marsh, J.L., Kraemer, B.B., Rayne, S.C., Gado, M.H., Moran, C.J., Mcalister, W.H., Shackelford, G.D., Hardesty, R.A.: Craniosynostosis: diagnostic imaging with three-dimensional CT presentation. Am. J. Neuroradiol. **15**, 1861–1869 (1994)

Towards a Statistical Shape-Aware Deformable Contour Model for Cranial Nerve Identification

Sharmin Sultana[1], Praful Agrawal[2], Shireen Y. Elhabian[2],
Ross T. Whitaker[2], Tanweer Rashid[1], Jason E. Blatt[3], Justin S. Cetas[4],
and Michel A. Audette[1(✉)]

[1] Department of MSVE, Old Dominion University, Norfolk, USA
{ssult003, trash001, maudette}@odu.edu
[2] Scientific Computing and Imaging Institute, University of Utah,
Salt Lake City, USA
{prafulag, whitaker}@cs.utah.edu,
shireen@sci.utah.edu
[3] Department of Neurosurgery and Radiology,
University of North Carolina, Chapel Hill, USA
jason.blatt@unchealth.unc.edu
[4] Department of Neurosurgery,
Oregon Health and Science University, Portland, USA
cetasj@ohsu.edu

Abstract. This paper presents a cranial nerve segmentation technique that combines a 3D deformable contour and a 3D contour Statistical Shape Model (SSM). A set of training data for the construction of the 3D contour shape model is produced using a 1-simplex based discrete deformable contour model where the centerline identification proceeds by optimizing internal and external forces. Point-correspondence for the training dataset is performed using an entropy-based energy minimization of particles on the centerline curve. The resulting average shape is used as *a prior* knowledge, which is incorporated into the 1-simplex as a reference shape model, making the approach stable against low resolution and image artifacts during segmentation using MRI data. Shape variability is shown using the first 3 modes of variation. The segmentation result is validated quantitatively, with ground truth provided by an expert.

Keywords: Cranial nerves · Centerline · Statistical Shape Model · Contour model · Patient-specific segmentation

1 Introduction

There are twelve pairs of Cranial Nerves (CN I to XII) that control our sensory functions such as vision, hearing, smell and taste as well as several motor functions of the head and neck including facial expressions, eye movement, and so on. Cranial nerves are at great risk during neurosurgical procedures in the skull base area, and damage to them is associated with life-altering morbidity such as the loss of eyesight,

© Springer International Publishing AG 2016
R. Shekhar et al. (Eds.): CLIP 2016, LNCS 9958, pp. 68–76, 2016.
DOI: 10.1007/978-3-319-46472-5_9

hearing or facial paralysis. It is thus vital to identify cranial nerves in MRI data for the planning of neurosurgical procedures where these critical structures might be at risk and also where these are targeted in treating cranial nerve disorders. Moreover, it is also important to build neurosurgery simulators where cranial nerves are accurately represented, despite the challenges to their segmentation.

With the exception of our on-going work [1], there is a paucity of research dedicated to segmenting cranial nerves for clinical use, particularly from T_1 or T_2-weighted MRI data, although preliminary efforts to reconstruct nerves from MR-DTI, a modality that is not widespread. Existing whole brain segmentation tools and brain atlases either do not account for cranial nerves, or can only segment larger ones like the optic nerve (CN II).

Previously, we presented an algorithm suitable for segmenting nerve centerline using 1-simplex based discrete 3D deformable model [1], where we identified nerves from T2-weighted MRI data. In this paper, the existing methodology of nerve segmentation is extended by integrating a Statistical Shape Model (SSM) into it. The goal of an SSM is to capture the shape mean and variations of the structures of interest. Shape information such as the average shape is incorporated into the deformable model as a priori knowledge, which makes this approach more stable against local image artifacts and partial volume effects while identifying nerve centerlines in medical images. We are currently in the process of integrating shape second-order statistics into the deformable model; however this research is still underway.

Cranial nerves are tube-like structures emanating from the human brain, from the brainstem (III to XII) or from attachments superior to it (I, II). While there is a tree-like aspect to nerves as well, it is more visible outside the cranium, whereby we make the assumption of simple curves in the intracranial portion. Tubular structure segmentation algorithms featuring shape statistics found in the literature have been employed in blood vessel segmentations. Nain et al. [2] proposed a blood vessel segmentation technique that incorporates image statistics and shape information in a region-based active contour model. A shape-driven 2D segmentation technique is presented in [3] for segmenting the atrial wall in ultrasound images where a non-parametric intensity model is used for lumen representation instead of parametric active contours. In Tejos and Irarrazaval [4], 2-simplex surface meshes are combined with statistical shape knowledge through Diffusion Snakes which is then applied to segment the patellar cartilage.

The rest of the paper is organized as follows: Sect. 2 overviews the existing cranial nerve segmentation algorithm; Sect. 3 describes the construction of statistical shape model; segmentation results using the method is presented in Sect. 4 and Sect. 5 contains conclusions and future works.

2 Overview of the Existing Centerline Extraction Technique

In this section, an overview of our previously published method for extracting nerve centerline from MRI data is described [1]. This discrete model-based nerve centerline identification technique consists of two main steps:

(a) First, a geodesic path between user defined end points is computed from the preprocessed MRI data. The geodesic path is the initial guess for the nerve centerline.

Gaussian smoothing is used to remove noise from the MRI data. Furthermore, a vesselness filtering [5] is employed to create preprocessed images. Then the geodesic path is computed using front propagation oriented fast marching method [6].

(b) Subsequently, a 1-simplex mesh-based model is constructed and deformed to get the final nerve centerline. The 1-simplex is a 3D discrete modeling technique where each non-terminating vertex has a constant 2-connectivity [7]. It is a Newtonian model where the vertex motion is based on internal and external forces. The dynamic behavior of a vertex P_i is represented as in Eq. (1):

$$m\frac{d^2P_i}{dt^2} = -\gamma\frac{dP_i}{dt} + F_{int} + F_{ext} \tag{1}$$

where, m is the mass of the vertex, γ is the damping factor, F_{int} and F_{ext} are internal and external forces, respectively. The computed geodesic path is then represented using a 1-simplex mesh which is deformed using internal and external forces towards the actual centerline of the curve.

3   Construction of Statistical Shape Models

3.1   Image Dataset and Training Shape Representation

We constructed a Statistical Shape Model from 5 volumetric MRI datasets provided by the National Institutes of Health (NIH). These datasets are Balanced Fast Field Echo (BFFE) sequences of slice with spacing $0.3 \times 0.3 \times 0.4$ mm^3, dimension $256 \times 256 \times 220$, TR = 5.45 ms and TE = 2.175 ms. Each of the dataset is segmented using our, existing centerline extraction technique, resulting in a set of 5 training shapes. The user has the option to manually correct this segmented centerlines so that the segmentation error does not propagate from training dataset to the shape-based atlas.

Each training shape is represented as a point-based 1-simplex model which facilitates computation of shape average and variations as well as shape-based force functional.

3.2   Modeling Average Shape and Shape Variations

The goal of the deformable shape modeling is to construct models by learning the patterns of shape variability from a training set of images and then deforming the model within the target image to be segmented in a manner consistent with these statistics. A Statistical Shape Model (SSM) computes the mean shape and a number of modes of variation from a pool of the training data set.

One of the main difficulties of SSMs is to produce point correspondences accurately across training shapes. Early methods used manual localization, but this overhead is prohibitive in 3D. The choice of dynamic particle-based positioning of landmark points for Principal Component Analysis is motivated by the limitations of a manual selection approach, which is prevalent in the Statistical Shape Models literature. The manual approach does not scale to the number of landmarks needed for 3D structures and it suffers from poor repeatability, particularly in 3D where definitive tissue boundaries are more difficult to locate. In response to this requirement of the SSM community, Cates, Whitaker et al. proposed a non-parametric sampling approach based on a cost function that favors a compact ensemble representation for a family of smooth shapes as well as a uniform distribution on each shape [8].

ContourWorks, a software toolkit developed by University of Utah, is used to establish point correspondence and compute statistical shape model for the training dataset. The objective function to be optimized is comprised of a cotangent-based sampling entropy [9] and covariance-based correspondence entropy [8]. The first term drives the sampling of points over the entire object boundary such that the shape of object is well represented by the set of points. The second term ensures a compact model in the shape space so that the control points in the final model corresponds geometrically across shapes in the training dataset. The 1-simplex nerve centerlines extracted from the MRI data are modeled using a set of points with each index point corresponding to same feature across the shape population.

Once the point correspondence is achieved, the next step is Shape Alignment. Since shapes are invariant under a similarity transform, training shapes need to be aligned by filtering out all the global transformations such as translation, scaling and rotation. The General Procrustes Analysis (GPA) is used for shape alignment, which iteratively aligns shapes by registering their corresponding point sets.

When all the shapes are brought into a common frame of reference, the modes that best describe the shape variations within that frame can be computed using Principle Component Analysis (PCA).

4   Shape Model-Based Segmentation

We used first order statistics such as the average shape model to identify nerve centerlines in MRI data. *First*, we find a minimal path from user identified start and end points which act as a rough estimation of the nerve's centerline. We used the Fast Marching method to compute the Minimal Path [6], based on the optimization of a cost functional defined from an image-based speed function. *Second*, the minimal path is then registered with the average shape model using a similarity transformation method. The transformed average shape is then used as a reference shape model to generate shape-based internal forces which is integrated into the 1-simplex during model deformation. From the transformed average shape we compute reference shape parameters $\left(\tilde{\varepsilon}_{1i}, \tilde{\varepsilon}_{2i}, \tilde{\phi}_i \text{ and } \tilde{\psi}_i \right)$ as in [10]. The average shape-based force is then calculated employing these reference shape parameters using Eq. (2)

$$F_{Shape} = \tilde{\varepsilon}_{1i}P_{N_1(i)} + \tilde{\varepsilon}_{2i}P_{N_2(i)} + h\left(\tilde{\phi}_i \right) n\left(\tilde{\psi}_i \right) - P_i \qquad (2)$$

Here $P_{N_1(i)}$ and $P_{N_2(i)}$ are the two neighbors of P_i. P_i is the i-th point of the 1-simplex model that needs to be deformed. $\tilde{\varepsilon}_{1i}, \tilde{\varepsilon}_{2i}, \tilde{\phi}_i$ and $\tilde{\psi}_i$ are reference parameters calculated from the average shape. $h\left(\tilde{\phi}_i\right)$ is the height function and $n\left(\tilde{\psi}_i\right)$ is the normal function calculated using the average shape parameters [10].

Finally, the 1-simplex model of the minimal path is deformed by minimizing internal forces, image-based external force and the average shape force. Here, we enforce two internal forces – a tangential force and a Laplacian force whereas the external force is based on the vesselness image information [1].

5   Results

5.1   Mean Shape and Variance

We have constructed statistical shape models for the facial nerve (CN VII) shown in Fig. 1. Figure 1(a) shows all the 5 segmented nerve centerlines of the left CNVII. The average shape for the left CNVII is shown in Fig. 1(b).

Similarly, Fig. 1(c) and (d) show the SSM for the right CNVII. The mean shape and shape variations of $\pm\,3\sigma$ along the first three principle modes for both left and right CNVII is graphically illustrated in Fig. 2. In each shape, 20 points were chosen for correspondence. Each correspondence point in the final shape model is shown using different colored balls.

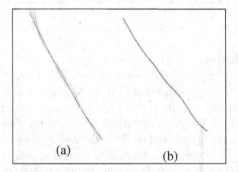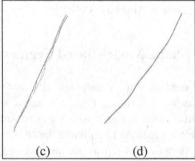

Fig. 1. Statistical Shape models for CNVII; (a) segmented left CNVIIs after shape alignment (shown in different colors); (b) The average shape of the left CNVII; (c) segmented right CNVIIs after shape alignment; (d) the average shape of the right CNVII;

For the shape model of the left CNVII, 4 modes of variation are able to capture 100 % of shape variations within the training dataset.

The shape model captured 65.26 % of variations within the 1st mode, 87.05 % within the 2nd mode, the 95.88 % within 3rd mode and 100 % of variability within 4th mode as shown in Fig. 2(a). On the other hand, only 3 modes of variation were able to capture 100 % shape variability of the training set as shown in the graph of Fig. 3(b).

5.2 Segmentation of Patient Data

We validated average shape models by segmenting a MRI data with partial volume effects. This MRI dataset was also provided by NIH. Although this dataset has the same voxel spacing of $0.3 \times 0.3 \times 0.4$ mm^3 like the training images, a few axial slices of CNVII has partial volume effects, as shown with the left red circle of Fig. 4(a). In this particular axial slice, even though CNVII has a clear appearance in right side as shown with the right red circle, it is not distinguishable very clearly in the left side.

CNVII originates from brainstem at the ventral part of the pontomedullary junction and exits through the internal auditory meatus. Two anatomical landmarks are placed at these end points by an expert, and these are used as the seed points in our method.

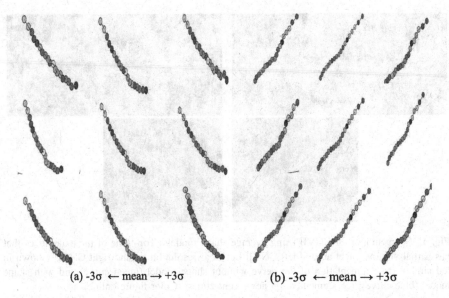

(a) -3σ ← mean → +3σ   (b) -3σ ← mean → +3σ

Fig. 2. Shape model variability: first 3 principal modes of (a) left and (b) right CNVII.

Figure 4 shows both the left and right part of the CNVII, segmented without using shape models (green curves) and segmented using our shape model (blue curves). In the case of the left side of CNVII, when the nerve is segmented without using shape models, the result is inaccurate for slices having partial volume effects because the image-based external forces fail to detect the nerve centerline in the presence of image artifacts. On the other hand, both segmentations (with and without shape models) show similar results for the right CNVII, as illustrated in Fig. 4.

A quantitative validation is performed by calculating error distances between the computed centerline using shape models and the ground truth centerline, as shown in Table 1. Mean distance and standard deviation are calculated from the points of computed centerlines to the curve of ground truth centerline whereas Hausdorff Distance is computed in a point-to-point fashion as shown in Fig. 5. The ground truth

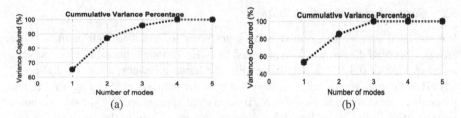

Fig. 3. Shape variability vs. number of modes of the constructed shape models. 100 % shape variations were captured within (a) first 4 modes of left CNVII shape model (b) first 3 modes of right CNVII shape model.

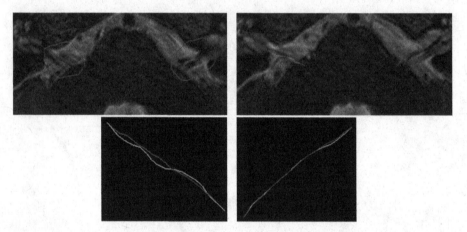

Fig. 4. Segmentation of CNVII using average shape models. Top- One of the axial slices that has partial volume effect around left CNVII but clear resolution around right CNVII (shown in red circle); (b) Segmentation of the nerve without shape model (green curve) and with shape model (blue curve); (c) segmented 3D nerve centerlines. (Color figure online)

Table 1. Quantitative validation of the shape-model based segmentation

	Mean distance (mm)	Std. deviation (mm)	Hausdorff Distance (mm)
Left CNVII	0.2649	0.1252	0.452
Right CNVII	0.1646	0.0985	0.313

centerline is a piecewise-linear path through a set of landmarks, manually provided by a neurosurgeon at UNC School of medicine, Chapel Hill NC.

The mean distance error is 0.2649 mm for the left CNVII and 0.1646 mm for the right. The standard deviation for the left CNVII is 12.52 % and 9.85 % for the right. The Hausdroff Distance measures how far the two segmentations are from each other and therefore quantitatively represents a measure of the worst segmentation error. The Hausdroff Distance, HD between two sets of points P and Q can be defined as $HD(P,Q) = max\{h(P,Q), h(Q,P)\}$, where $h(A,B) = max_{a \in A}\{min_{b \in B}\{d(a,b)\}\}$.

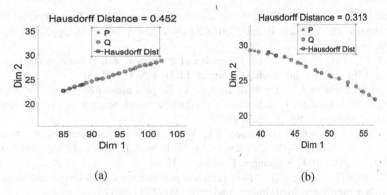

Fig. 5. Graphical representation of Hausdroff Distance between computed centerlines (marked by red o) and ground-truth centerlines (marked by blue x): (a) left CNVII (b) right CNVII. (Color figure online)

The Hausdroff Distance for the left CNVII is 0.452 and 0.313 for the right, as graphically shown in Fig. 5.

6 Conclusion and Future Works

A statistical shape driven deformable model-based cranial nerve segmentation technique has been described in this paper. 5 MRI datasets are used for identifying cranial nerves using the existing 1-simplex deformable model [1], which are used as the training dataset for the construction of the shape model. The computed shape models can faithfully capture 100 % shape variations within the population using a maximum of 4 modes of variation. The segmentation of a specific cranial nerve (CNVII) is shown in this paper with encouraging results. Nerve centerlines were delineated accurately from a MRI dataset with the presence of partial volume effects.

One limitation in this paper is the use of a small training dataset. Accuracy would be improved when using a larger dataset, which should be able to capture larger variations of the sample population. Another limitation is the fact that we have used only first order statistics (average shape) for the shape model-based segmentation. We are currently working on incorporating shape covariance into the shape-based force.

References

1. Sultana, S., Blatt, J.E., Lee, Y., Ewend, M., Cetas, J.S., Costa, A., Audette, M.A.: Patient-specific cranial nerve identification using a discrete deformable contour model for skull base neurosurgery planning and simulation. In: Oyarzun Laura, C., et al. (eds.) CLIP 2015. LNCS, vol. 9401, pp. 36–44. Springer, Heidelberg (2016). doi:10.1007/978-3-319-31808-0_5

2. Nain, D., Yezzi, A.J., Turk, G.: Vessel segmentation using a shape driven flow. In: Barillot, C., Haynor, D.R., Hellier, P. (eds.) MICCAI 2004. LNCS, vol. 3216, pp. 51–59. Springer, Heidelberg (2004)

3. Unal, G., et al.: Shape-driven segmentation of the arterial wall in intravascular ultrasound images. IEEE Trans. Inf. Technol. Biomed. **12**(3), 335–347 (2008)

4. Tejos, C., Irarrazaval, P., Cárdenas-Blanco, A.: Simplex mesh diffusion snakes: integrating 2D and 3D deformable models and statistical shape knowledge in a variational framework. Int. J. Comput. Vis. **85**(1), 19–34 (2009)

5. Frangi, A.F., Niessen, W.J., Vincken, K.L., Viergever, M.A.: Multiscale vessel enhancement filtering. In: Wells, W.M., Colchester, A.C.F., Delp, S.L. (eds.) MICCAI 1998. LNCS, vol. 1496, pp. 130–137. Springer, Heidelberg (1998)

6. Deschamps, T., Cohen, L.D.: Fast extraction of minimal paths in 3D images and applications to virtual endoscopy. Med. Image Anal. **5**(4), 281–299 (2001)

7. Delingette, H.: General object reconstruction based on simplex meshes. Int. J. Comput. Vis. **32**(2), 111–146 (1999)

8. Cates, J.E., Fletcher, P.T., Styner, M.A., Shenton, M.E., Whitaker, R.T.: Shape modeling and analysis with entropy-based particle systems. In: Karssemeijer, N., Lelieveldt, B. (eds.) IPMI 2007. LNCS, vol. 4584, pp. 333–345. Springer, Heidelberg (2007)

9. Meyer, M.D., Georgel, P., Whitaker, R.T.: Robust particle systems for curvature dependent sampling of implicit surfaces. In: International Conference on Shape Modeling and Applications. IEEE (2005)

10. Gilles, B., Magnenat-Thalmann, N.: Musculoskeletal MRI segmentation using multi-resolution simplex meshes with medial representations. Med. Image Anal. **14**(3), 291–302 (2010)

An Automatic Free Fluid Detection for Morrison's-Pouch

Matthias Noll[1,2]([⊠]) and Stefan Wesarg[1,2]

[1] Fraunhofer IGD, Darmstadt, Germany
{matthias.noll,stefan.wesarg}@igd.fraunhofer.de
[2] GRIS, Technische Universität Darmstadt, Darmstadt, Germany
http://s.fhg.de/vht

Abstract. Ultrasound provides a useful and readily available imaging tool to detect free fluids in blunt abdominal trauma patients. However, applying conventional 2D ultrasound to diagnose the patient requires a well trained physician. In this paper we describe a fully automatic free fluid detection pipeline for the hepathorenal recess or Morrison's pouch using 3D ultrasound acquisitions. The image data is collected using the standardized "Focused Assessment with Sonography for Trauma" (FAST) exam. Our method extracts key structures like the kidney and the liver from the image data and uses their relative positions to search and detect free fluids between the organ interfaces. To evaluate our method we have developed a free fluid simulation that allows us to generate free fluid images using acquisitions of healthy volunteers. Our intentions are to enable even untrained ultrasound operators to perform a free fluid diagnosis of an injured person. In order to do this, our method additionally provides basic image acquisition guidance information.

Keywords: Ultrasound · Free fluid · Trauma · Kidney · Liver · Segmentation

1 Introduction

Abdominal trauma is one of the major injury patterns in modern society. In [2] a collective of 300 trauma patients was examined. Of those, 248 (or 82.6 %) did exhibit some form of abdominal trauma. With 69.4 % the majority of the abdominal trauma patients presented with non-penetrating blunt force abdominal trauma (BAT). The reason for this is, that modern and better safety mechanisms increasingly protect the body from being penetrated, but the shear forces that can arise can cause BAT, regardlessly. BAT patients suffer from invisible internal hemorrhaging that if undetected can lead to death within only a few hours. Therefore, immediate and continues medical care for BAT patients is indispensable. Unfortunately, internal injuries can be hard to detect during the initial exam because the patient may not show any visible trauma signs.

There are two major imaging modalities of choice that allow the diagnosis of internal hemorrhaging in form of free fluids, which accumulate in body cavities.

© Springer International Publishing AG 2016
R. Shekhar et al. (Eds.): CLIP 2016, LNCS 9958, pp. 77–84, 2016.
DOI: 10.1007/978-3-319-46472-5_10

The more sensitive and stationary CT or the portable, not harmful and readily available ultrasound. Usually the CT is located inside the hospital in a separate shielded room and it's operated by trained radiologists who are also able to properly interpret the generated images. Here, the benefits and need for automatic CT based free fluid detection algorithms are negligible. However, enabling ultrasound devices to achieve automatic free fluid detection may generate huge benefits, because a portable ultrasound can pretty much be operated anywhere and by anybody with access to the device (e.g. an EMT). This could even be an untrained person who is far away from the next hospital.

Apart from its benefits, ultrasound has some major challenges. The biggest challenge is, that the ultrasound transducer must be positioned at the correct body location and it must point to the examination target with the exact scan angle. This especially applies for the examination of the right upper quadrant (RUQ) view of the FAST exam [3], that is conducted through the ribs and visualizes Morrison's-pouch. The ribs cause shadowing artefact's that can occlude important image information like the free fluid region. For this reason, the exam is usually performed by a trained physician. The main challenge of performing an ultrasound exam originates in the limited field of view of conventional 2D ultrasound transducers. The 2D ultrasound plane must be perfectly aligned with the target structure and even then, the sonographer applies panning shots to see all surrounding elements of the target. This limitation can be reduced by applying 3D ultrasound. The essential advantage over 2D ultrasound is that a complete volume of the patients anatomy is recorded during a single acquisition.

Applying 3D ultrasound in combination with 3D image processing algorithms, an untrained operator would only require some basic information about where to place the probe on the patients body. This placement can then be optimized by deriving guidance informations for the operator, directly from the image content. We will describe in Sect. 2.1 how this can be achieved. Luckily, trauma protocols like the FAST exam already define a standardized probe placement for the important free fluid accumulation regions, thus it is a perfect staring point for an automatic approach.

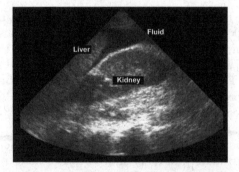

Fig. 1. 2D ultrasound of Morrison's pouch showing the kidney, the liver and the anechoic free fluid region.

2   Methods

There are basically two approaches how free fluids can be detected. The first approach is to apply some form of image processing method to the image e.g. thresholding. This approach usually does not require any additional context or model information. However, this approach does also not consider, that many fluids inside the body won't be free fluids. For instance, the entire vascular system as well as organs like the bladder or the heart do contain or transport allot of contained fluids. Additionally, artifacts like ultrasound shadows and other disruptive influences as speckle may complicate the detection even further. The second approach utilizes context information that may be derived from the image and adapts the following scanning paradigm of physicians:

1. Detect a landmark that is specific for the target location
2. Start the search for abnormalities form there

In the remaining sections of this paper we follow the latter approach and exploit the volumetric ultrasound information to achieve the fluid detection.

2.1   The RUQ Approach Using Landmarks

Since we apply the FAST exam to acquire the RUQ view, we need to detect a landmark that is characteristic for the Morrison's-Pouch view. We know that the RUQ image contains the kidney and the liver. The kidney is relatively small compared to the liver and can fit entirely into the image volume. The liver in contrast is way too large to fit inside a single volume. Therefore, we use the kidney as the landmark for the free fluid search. Choosing the kidney also has some advantages. The biggest advantage is, that we do not require any image processing if the kidney is not detected. The operator must tilt the probe until the kidney is within the image. Only then the algorithm will continue. Another important advantage is that once the probe is placed at the correct position, we can inform the operator where the kidney was detected in the volume. This again can be used to calculate adjustment angles α and β to optimize the transducer tilt, so that the kidney will move e.g. to the volume center. The angles can be calculated as the rotational component between the target vector $\overrightarrow{t_c k_c}$ from the transducer center t_c to the kidney center k_c and the image x and z axis.

The kidney detection can be achieved using one of the methods in [1,4,8,9]. In our setup we perform the kidney detection using the algorithm described in [9]. Once the kidney location is found, we apply a model based kidney segmentation method to extract the kidney region. The implementation of the kidney segmentation is based on [7,10] and is similar to the approach of [8]. However, it won't be discussed further in this paper.

Because Morrison's-Pouch is located between the liver and the kidney, the next natural step is to extract the liver. Optimally, we would like to segment the entire liver to establish the location of Morrison's pouch. Sadly, this is not easy because most of the liver surface is outside the volume or can't be easily recognized. Also the liver tissue intensity is rarely uniform to be easily segmented.

The only practical liver features are the vessel structures. Segmenting the liver vessel tree provides the skeletal structure for at least a small liver region. Still, even with a small liver region we can determine the fluid search vector and validate the correct RUQ view acquisition. In our approach we performed the vessel extraction analogue to [6], while placing the required seed points automatically at the highest vesselness values. The ultrasound resolution only allows to detect lager vessels inside the organ. With this in mind we can argue that only liver tissue will be found between the extracted vessel structures. Thus, we can simply generate a convex hull from the vessel structures to obtain a small chunk of the liver region. We have not further investigated a more complete liver segmentation because we don't require a larger liver region at this point.

2.2   Free Fluid Simulation

It is not easy to obtain ultrasound images of BAT patients with free fluids in the RUQ. It is even harder to acquire suitable 3D ultrasound images, because the technology is not yet as common in trauma medicine as it is e.g. in gynaecology. Therefore, we have implemented a free fluid generator that takes a user specified region and a free fluid intensity range $[I_{min}, I_{max}]$ as its input and applies both to an arbitrary real ultrasound image to simulate a free fluid like region. The user specified region serves as a mask for the ultrasound. It's pixels are randomly filled with the provided intensity values $I \in [I_{min}, I_{max}]$. To produce a more realistic appearance of the region, the generator also applies morphological dilatation and erosion operations to generate a corona around the fluid mask. The corona is then filled with high and low intensity values based on the angular intensity function (1), where the utilized constants correlate to ratio of the golden section. The required angles are derived using the mask center m_c and the corona pixel p_c by calculating $\angle(\overrightarrow{m_c p_c}, \overrightarrow{y})$ the angle between the direction vector $\overrightarrow{m_c p_c}$ and the ultrasound scan direction, which is equal to the images' y axis. This is an attempt to simulate the directionality of the ultrasound response.

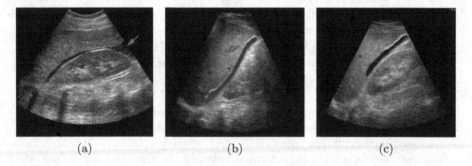

(a)   (b)   (c)

Fig. 2. Image (a) shows real free fluid in the RUQ. The free fluid simulation with different parameters for α_{max} and fluid intensity range (b) and (c).

$$f(\alpha) = \begin{cases} 0 & \text{if } \alpha > \alpha_{max} \\ 255 * \frac{\alpha}{\alpha_{max}} * 0,618 + 0,382 & \text{otherwise} \end{cases} \tag{1}$$

The corona region is further dilated to twice its original size to fill some occurring holes. The simulation is finalized by applying some Gaussian smoothing on the corona. Two simulation results are shown in Fig. 2 where they can be compared to an ultrasound with real free fluids.

2.3 Fluid Detection and Segmentation

For the fluid detection, it is important to know that both the liver and the kidney or just one of them may not be found. The reasons for this can be manifold, thus we need to apply certain algorithmic steps that will still assure the free fluid detection. We could test for both organs initially, but a vessel detection does not automatically imply that the liver is detected. In a high resolution ultrasound the kidney vessels are also visible and produce strong vesselness signals as well. Hence, we have chosen not to detect the liver early on. The kidney as our algorithms reference structure must be detected, regardlessly. Otherwise the algorithm does not continue. For a positive kidney detection, we can still search along the organ boundaries for free fluids. However, having both organ regions is the ideal case. We can search the area between the organs along the search vector $v_s = l_c - k_c$ with the liver vessels' convex hull center l_c and the kidney center k_c (see Fig. 3a). We do this for all surface points facing the liver. If the liver is not detected, we need to search in the direction of the transducer origin. At this point we must assume, that the image was acquired using FAST and that it shows the organs at the correct location. Otherwise we need to search along the entire kidney surface. The search vector without a detected liver can be set as $v_s = u_c - k_c$ with u_c being the ultrasound transducer center and the kidney center k_c. As can be seen in Fig. 3b, we extend the search range to include all surface normals of the kidney that deviate about 30–60 degrees from the search vectors' direction.

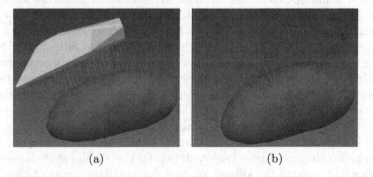

(a)   (b)

Fig. 3. The free fluid search from kidney to liver using direct search vectors (a) and the extended search for free fluids with no detected liver region (b).

Along the search direction, we apply the local entropy criterion from [5] to detect strong "signal ruptures", that are caused by the transition from tissue to the fluid region. This is done iteratively for all search vectors to generate seed points for the free fluid segmentation. As the fluid region will separate the liver and kidney interface, a search along v_s should produce two strong signal ruptures, one for the start and one for the end of the fluid region. We place the seed point in the middle of the first two strong signal ruptures. A search line is discarded, when less than two ruptures are detected.

After the seed point generation we apply a region growing method to extract the free fluid region. The result of the free fluid search and segmentation can be observed in Fig. 4 for both 2D and 3D.

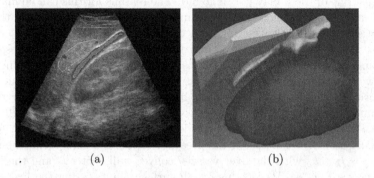

(a)   (b)

Fig. 4. The free fluid detection and segmentation result. Image (a) shows the result in the 2D standard plane. Image (b) is the 3D visualization of the search from the kidney (red) to the liver region (yellow) applying both search strategies. The fluid region is visualized in cyan in the middle of both organ regions.

3   Results

Our evaluation data is composed of 30 3D ultrasound volumes of the RUQ FAST view. Additionally we have a single 4D data set of a moving kidney that includes 31 ultrasound volumes. The datasets with an extend of $177 \times 249 \times 177$ pixels were collected using a GE Voluson E ultrasound device. The kidney center was successfully detected in 55 cases, which is a detection rate of 90,16 %. The cause for the failed detections were either that the kidney cortex and pelvis were covered by a rib shadow or that the kidney cortex was detected next to the liver at the kidney interface. This is a problem of the chosen detection method [9]. The former was the case for 4 volumes, the latter for 2 volumes. Nonetheless, the initialization of the model-based segmentation was still possible with the falsely detected kidney position at the liver border. Thus, we could extract the kidney region applying the model-based segmentation for the remaining 26 datasets with a detection in or around the kidney. We have evaluated our segmentation results against 20 available expert segmentations, which yielded a DICE coefficient of $\mu = 0.8147$ with a standard deviation of $\sigma = 0.0656$.

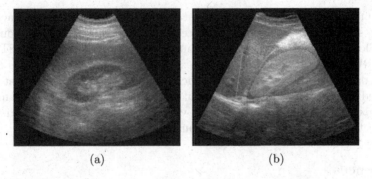

(a)   (b)

Fig. 5. The 4D data slice (a) does not shows any visible vessel structures in kidney or liver. Image (b) shows an overlap between the extracted kidney and the liver region as a result of too low vesselness values in the liver.

Besides the kidney, we were able to detect and extract the liver region in 27 of 30 cases (90 %). We did not use the 4D dataset for the liver detection because the volumes do not contain any visible vessel structures (cf. Fig. 5a). In the 3 datasets without a valid liver region the calculated vesselness values were not strong enough to point to the liver region. Instead, the automatically extracted vessels were partially or completely located inside the kidney region Fig. 5b. In this case the free fluid detection failed, as the direction vector did not pass the simulated fluid region. Though, this case is easy to detect by calculating the intersection set of both segmentations, which must be empty. To resolve this issue, all vessels inside the segmented kidney region can be removed from the image. Additionally, the liver detection could be discarded, defaulting the search to the second approach without the liver. We have simulated the fluid region for 10 datasets, with and without the liver region. The detection was successful in all cases.

4   Discussion

We have proposed a method to determine the free fluid status of the RUQ view of the FAST exam. To achieve the free fluid search, we have extracted the kidney region as the algorithms reference structure. Additionally, we have extracted a liver region by exploiting the vessel structures as liver features. The detection of free fluids was performed between both organ regions in the Morrison's pouch. The algorithm does cope with a failed liver detection by applying an additional search strategy. The fluid segmentation was achieved through region growing on automatically placed seed points. Due to the difficult nature of obtaining appropriate 3D ultrasound images of the RUQ with free fluids we have implemented a free fluid simulation tool to generate our testing data from the available datasets. Using these images we have shown the validity of our approach. To our knowledge our algorithm is the first attempt of automatically detecting free fluids in 3D ultrasound data of Morrison's pouch applying the FAST exam. The benefit of our approach is, that the 3D image data allows the simultaneous extraction of multiple structures to determine the free fluid location. Furthermore, our approach allows users who are not ultrasound experts to perform the FAST exam for the RUQ. Future work will include extensive tests of our algorithms on real trauma datasets. This work will also include a more precise assessment of the extracted fluid region. Additionally, we like to expand our algorithmic framework to incorporate the left upper quadrant view (LUQ) of the FAST exam, which can directly benefit from components our presented algorithm.

References

1. Ardon, R., Cuingnet, R., Bacchuwar, K., Auvray, V.: Fast kidney detection and segmentation with learned kernel convolution and model deformation in 3d ultrasound images. In: 2015 IEEE 12th International Symposium on Biomedical Imaging (ISBI), pp. 268–271, April 2015
2. Gad, M.A., Saber, A., Farrag, S., Shams, M.E., Ellabban, G.M.: Incidence, patterns, and factors predicting mortality of abdominal injuries in trauma patients. North Am. J. Med. Sci. **4**(3), 129–34 (2012)
3. Rozycki, G.S., Ochsner, M.G., Feliciano, D.V., Thomas, B., Boulanger, B.R., Davis, F.E., Falcone, R.E., Schmidt, J.A.: Early detection of hemoperitoneum by ultrasound examination of the right upper quadrant: a multicenter study. J. Trauma. **45**(5), 878–883 (1998)
4. Hafizah, W.M., Supriyanto, E.: Automatic region of interest generation for kidney ultrasound images. In: Proceedings of the 11th WSEAS International Conference on Applied Computer Science, pp. 70–75, ACS 2011, World Scientific and Engineering Academy and Society (WSEAS), Stevens Point, Wisconsin, USA (2011)
5. Hellier, P., Coupe, P., Meyer, P., Morandi, X., Collins, D.: Acoustic shadows detection, application to accurate reconstruction of 3d intraoperative ultrasound. In: 5th IEEE International Symposium on Biomedical Imaging: from Nano to Macro, 2008, ISBI 2008, pp. 1569–1572 (2008)
6. Keil, M., Laura, C.O., Drechsler, K., Wesarg, S.: Combining B-mode and color flow vessel segmentation for registration of hepatic CT and ultrasound volumes. In: Ropinski, T., Ynnerman, A., Botha, C., Roerdink, J. (eds.) Eurographics Workshop on Visual Computing for Biology and Medicine. The Eurographics Association (2012)
7. Kirschner, M.: The probabilistic active shape model: from model construction to flexible medical image segmentation. Ph.D. thesis, TU Darmstadt (2013)
8. Marsousi, M., Plataniotis, K., Stergiopoulos, S.: Shape-based kidney detection and segmentation in three-dimensional abdominal ultrasound images. In: Engineering in Medicine and Biology Society (EMBC), 2014 36th Annual International Conference of the IEEE, pp. 2890–2894, August 2014
9. Noll, M., Nadolny, A., Wesarg, S.: Automated kidney detection for 3d ultrasound using scan line searching (2016)
10. Steger, S., Kirschner, M., Wesarg, S.: Articulated atlas for segmentation of the skeleton from head amp; neck ct datasets. In: 2012 9th IEEE International Symposium on Biomedical Imaging (ISBI), pp. 1256–1259, May 2012

Author Index

Printed in the United States
By Bookmasters